THE

Potty Training Answer Book

Practical Answers to the Top 200 Questions Parents Ask

KAREN DEERWESTER

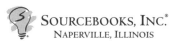

SOURCEBOOKS, INC.®
NAPERVILLE, ILLINOIS

D1377115

Published by Sourcebooks, Inc.
P.O. Box 4410, Naperville, Illinois 60567-4410
(630) 961-3900
Fax: (630) 961-2168
www.sourcebooks.com

Printed and bound in the United States of America.
VP 10 9 8 7 6 5 4 3 2 1

Dedication

To parents everywhere who never give up,
May your bathrooms be happy places.
And to Amanda, Brett, and Ayden,
The love keeps growing.

Contents

Acknowledgments

This book was written with the help of thousands of parents who shared their stories and their children's early years with me. Some of their one-time two-year-olds have now graduated from college. I cherish the times we laughed and sometimes cried together, continually celebrating the magical world of young children. Thank you for showing me the joys and the struggles of parenthood. Our time together will always be among the greatest gifts in my life.

A special thank-you goes to the staff and families of the Ruth and Edward Taubman Early Childhood Center at B'nai Torah Congregation of Boca Raton. Your potty training questions kept me writing when I wondered if I had said all there was to say. Thank you to Pam Appelbaum, Heather Mesch, Leesa Parker, Adele Weissblatt, and Amy Weissman for encouraging me while patiently reading sections for this book. You never ran the other way when I approached you for help. Thank you to Rabbi David Steinhardt, Rabbi David Englander, Rabbi Amy

Rader, Stephen Lippy, and especially Nancy Goldstein for inviting Family Time into your amazing school and your joyful community. I feel very fortunate to have a Mommy and Me home at B'nai Torah Congregation.

A heartfelt thank-you goes to María Bailey, for continually inspiring me to try new things; Dr. Michelle LaRocque, for taking the time to lend her early childhood knowledge and professional feedback; Dr. Jordan Mussary, MD, FAAP, for reviewing the pediatrician's list; and Bethany Brown at Sourcebooks, Inc., for her detailed insights, her optimism, and her belief that I was the right person for this project.

Thank you to all the other friends and family who keep me smiling. To Paula Basa, Louise Goldberg, Ellyn Laub, Tim Leistner, Ellen Munnelly, Liza Muschett, and Joan Stillwell—thanks for keeping me on schedule, for allowing my writing to interrupt more important things you may have been doing, and for sustaining friendships that are bigger than a book and so much bigger than today. To Dave Sestrich, thanks for standing by me through thick and thin. Thanks to Lynn and Heather for cheering for me. And finally, thanks to Richard. I couldn't have gotten to this point in my life without you. You showed me how to have big dreams. I love you all very much.

Introduction

Your child is a unique little person with a blooming personality. He is ready, or nearly ready, to embark on one of the greatest adventures of early childhood— learning to control his body and potty in a special place. He is ready, or nearly ready, to know what he needs and to manage some unique potty situations.

He has no idea why this is a big deal to so many people around him. He does not know that so many people will be watching and waiting to hear about his potty progress. He does not know some people expect him to do this a certain way or in a specific amount of time. Luckily, he has no idea others think he can fail.

Your child cannot fail.
All children are potty trained in good time. Naturally, there are obstacles and setbacks, and potty training rarely goes the way you imagine. However, if you are prepared and realistic about your child and your situation, potty training is a fun and positive experience. You will not fail.

Potty training is a natural step in development. Your child has been growing at incredible speed for the last few years. Just as she learned to walk, talk, sing, dance, climb, and laugh, she now wants to take care of her body. Just as she learned to imitate, pretend, be serious, and be silly, she now wants to learn more and do more. Although it felt great for a while to have someone else meeting all of her needs, she now realizes the satisfaction and joy of acting on her own. The first time your toddler looked at you and said, "No," your little girl began her growth toward independence.

Potty training is an inevitable rite of passage for you and your child. Together you will learn to use developmental skills to accomplish a task that signals a move from one stage of dependency to a new stage of independence. You and your child are growing. Shout "Hooray!"

This book will be by your side, answering each and every question that arises during your personal potty training adventure. You will know what potty training readiness looks like. You will know how to prepare your child for potty training. You will know how to make the transition from diapers to a potty and to support any possible confusion or resistance.

However, a one-size potty plan does not fit all potty training situations. Your potty training experiences will be just as unique as you and your child. This book will help you to customize the perfect plan for your child with a full awareness of your child's personal strengths and complete respect for your child's individuality. Your child is never "wrong" for doing things his way. Your personal potty plan celebrates your child and his childhood while giving you and your child the tools to move forward with confidence.

Come along—take this potty adventure knowing that you will be successful. Listen and watch your child. This is his time to discover everything he can do. This is your time to follow where he wants to go and to lead him to places he never imagined.

You can read this book by jumping to the questions that meet your immediate needs or you can read through the questions chapter by chapter. Each chapter moves you deeper into the day-to-day reality of potty training.

Whatever your potty experience, congratulations on reaching this point. In time you can say, "I did it!"

Chapter 1

POTTY TRAINING BASICS

- Does potty training mean different things to different people?
- What are some popular potty training theories?
- What is a potty training myth and what is reality?
- Is a potty training method ever wrong for my child?
- Can I borrow different strategies from different theories?
- Is consistency important?
- Do disposable diapers change the potty training experience?
- How else is potty training different now than in past generations?
- Do preschool requirements make potty training more difficult?
- What is the average age for children to be potty trained?
- Is it possible to potty train babies under one year old?
- Do girls potty train earlier than boys?
- Do boys potty train sitting down or standing up?
- Are second children easier to potty train?
- Does peer pressure make potty training easier?
- What is potty training etiquette in public situations?
- Which comes first—potty training for pee or for poop?
- How do I teach the proper way to wipe after pottying?

- Is there anything I should do before my child is ready for potty training?
- What advantages are there to potty training earlier?
- What advantages are there to potty training later?
- Is it possible to wait too long to start potty training?
- How does potty training affect self-esteem?
- Is potty training different in different cultures?

Does potty training mean different things to different people?

Potty training can mean many different things, although they all lead to the same outcome—your child's understanding and control of his body. The methods may differ drastically or the methods may be interchangeable and complementary. Some people believe potty training is a natural process that is easily learned at the right time, while others believe it is urgently taught with very specific adult intervention. Unfortunately, in many cases potty training feels like a dreadful chore.

The underlying truth is that all children enjoy taking control of their bodies. And all parents have the ability to make potty learning a positive and even fun experience. Children want to grow up as long as change is safe and manageable. You want to support your child through each developmental stage—cultivating skills, encouraging through failures, and designing winning solutions.

Different potty training strategies will work for different families at different times. While the basics will be true for all children, sometimes a specific shortcut will get you over the hump in a frustrating situation. There is always a solution to help you and your child move forward.

What are some popular potty training theories?

Infant potty training
In many cultures around the world, potty training begins with children under one year of age. Organizations like DiaperFreeBaby have recently described "elimination communication" as a natural family philosophy consistent with their interpretation of attachment parenting. Mom, or another caregiver, is a full-time participant in the pottying process: timing feedings and eliminations, reading baby's physical cues, and holding the baby on the potty. Proponents of this method believe it saves on diaper costs, minimizes environmental waste, and leads to deep parent–child bonding. It is also time-intensive and can only be done in an emotionally supportive environment.

Dr. Sears' Attachment Parenting

Attachment parenting celebrates emotional and physical bonding between parents and children through breast-feeding, co-sleeping, and responsive intimacy. In Dr. Sears' book *You Can Go to the Potty*, he describes potty training as potty learning. The learning process is a natural progression toward independence through loving parental support. Children are fed, rocked to sleep, and diapered by grown-ups. Then, as children grow and learn language, they choose to eat, sleep, and potty on their own.

Potty training in a day

This method accelerates potty training by increasing fluid intake and thereby increasing potty opportunities. It is recommended for children over twenty months old if both parents are in agreement. Readiness conditions should be apparent for the child to begin. In this method, children learn about the pottying process by teaching a doll that wets and using a reward system that reinforces the child's success. Parental approval and disapproval are intended to lead the child to the desired behaviors.

American Academy of Pediatrics

The American Academy of Pediatrics (AAP) guidelines focus on a positive developmental approach to potty training. The guidelines recognize a range of ages to begin potty training based on differences in readiness factors and family dynamic. The AAP recommendations are individualized and allow for months from beginning to mastery.

"No Pants" Toilet Training

In this method, the diaper is removed as an obstacle to children feeling the physical sensations of pottying. The method presupposes the other readiness factors are in place. It may also be a method suitable for some children with special needs, in that it gently yet directly teaches about the potty process. Parents, or caregivers, simplify the child's schedule and focus attention on learning the new potty experience.

What is a potty training myth and what is reality?

One parent's truth can easily be another parent's myth. Imagine parenting choices to be a long buffet table filled with recipes made from land, sea, and air prepared in dozens of different ways from deep fried to steamed. Then add seasonings from all around the world. Some will be your favorites. Some you will love to eat but regret in the morning. There will be those that your best friend would die for, even though you wouldn't taste it if someone paid you. Just to confuse things a little more, there will be dishes that you loved two years ago that just don't do it for you anymore.

Searching for the right potty training strategy is just like that. You have many choices, and your friends will swear by the strategy that worked for them. Scan the buffet. Try small tastes of the choices that you like. Before you know it, you will have a full plate of things that really work for you and your child at this particular time.

The myth is that there is one right way for every child. Children create the exceptions to every great theory. It doesn't take long to find out a certain food doesn't agree with you. Likewise, by the time you finish this book, you will know how to choose or modify potty training strategies that work for you.

Is a potty training method ever wrong for my child?

Yes, when potty training feels like a battle, it's wrong for your child. Remember, parents always lose power struggles because the rules of engagement are on the child's terms, not the adult's terms. If you feel a power struggle brewing, quickly call for an emotional truce. Give yourself a momentary time-out to regroup or consider a large scale re-evaluation of your plan.

Resistance comes in two forms: (1) the hesitant uncertainty of learning something new, confusing, and challenging; and (2) the dig-in-your-heels defiance of you-can't-make-me. The second form of resistance will not be productive to moving forward to potty training and requires a re-evaluation. If emotions are flying out of control—screaming, panicky coercion, blind desperation, or fearful anxiety— STOP! It's time to change course.

Some frustration, as in all learning situations, is natural. Potty teachers welcome the opportunity to build confidence and encourage a sense of "I can do it." You will witness your child's vulnerabilities and even some behavioral testing. But you and your child should always be on the same side and never at war with one another.

Can I borrow different strategies from different theories?

Finding a potty training strategy that doesn't need to be tweaked to fit your child is like bringing home a newborn that sleeps through the night. You can swear that it's because you did all the right things at the right time, but chances are your second child will prove that theory wrong.

Potty training is personal. You are learning about how your child learns and masters her body and her world. You are learning about yourself as a teacher—what frustrates you and what inspires you. Your child's potty training experiences involve trust, decision making, perseverance through mistakes, and the ability to conquer obstacles.

Any potty training program that minimizes the people factor in favor of a right method falls short. Some potty training situations require more creativity than others, and some children need more support than others. Focus on your child—she's not wrong just because she's not responding the right way. Feel free to make your modifications to any theory.

Is consistency important?

Yes, consistency is important. However, consistency is often preceded by a period of trial and error. Real world situations add unexpected challenges to the best laid plans.

Potty training takes both the parent and child into unknown territory, as each potty training experience is different from all others. Using the earlier example of the buffet of choices, you can't possibly know beforehand that eating a beautiful piece of chocolate cake will make you break out in hives. In the same way, trial and error is a legitimate parenting strategy to find what works and what doesn't.

As things click, you can build a consistent plan: foods and routines that make potty choices easier, the right motivating words, and small repeatable successes. Informed knowledge that is personal to your situation will become your child's familiar day-to-day experience. In this case, the potty experience is familiar, predictable, and non-threatening—something your child can control. If you are consistent with yourself, your child will understand what's expected of him.

Do disposable diapers change the potty training experience?

Children today aren't different from past generations of children, although the world around them is different. The biggest change is in the diaper industry. Children potty trained before disposable diapers (or who wore cloth diapers) could readily feel the effects of pooping and peeing in their diaper. Diapers got wet, droopy, and markedly heavy. The post-potty experience was distinct from the pre-potty experience, which easily motivated some children to experiment with holding their pee and poop to relieve in other places.

Diaper technology, however, whisked the wetness away from the body. Disposable diapers kept children feeling very comfortable, and kept moms happy that their babies were clean. Unfortunately, children lost the awareness of a classic physical discomfort.

Diaper companies soon found a solution to assist children in the potty training process even though they were still wearing disposable diapers. Some diapers change color when wet. This is good news for children who are more logical thinkers—"Ah, I see a change in color that means my body did something when I wasn't paying attention to it." Other diapers feel cold when wet. The sensation gives children immediate physical feedback of what their body is doing.

Once upon a time, diapers may have carried a stigma of being "for babies." Now, diapers have attractive characters for all diaper-wearing ages. Diapers aren't just diapers anymore, either. There are also "pull-ups" and "trainers" marketed for older toddlers and preschoolers. The good news is that this generation is less likely to humiliate children into becoming big boys and girls. The bad news is parents might not always be aware of mixed messages surrounding potty training.

How else is potty training different now than in past generations?

Family schedules are different now than in past generations. Family life is not as home-centric. The number of playgroups, Mommy and Me, music, and gymnastic classes for the pre-preschool set has grown significantly in the last twenty-five years. Babies are "on the go" long before their first birthday. By the time they approach their second birthday, their social calendar is often busier than that of their parents.

Potty training is either something to fit into an already busy day or requires a major hiatus in the schedule. These are deliberate choices that past generations never had to make.

Pressure is everywhere these days as parenthood becomes professionalized. Parents try to do their very best, especially in the critical early childhood years.

The Internet brings developmental, educational, and pediatric research to inquiring fingers everywhere. Today's parents face an information overload of unprecedented proportions. Community is no longer just the neighbor next door, but also parents in similar situations anywhere in the world. The global community brings you new connections but sometimes lacks the familiar supports of lifelong family and friends.

With all these changes, potty training remains something all young children will eventually master—and all parents will survive.

Do preschool requirements make potty training more difficult?

Preschools set policies about potty training according to each school's educational philosophy. You should discuss any concerns about your child's potty readiness prior to enrolling her. Most schools understand firsthand the process and problems associated with potty training. These schools will be able to evaluate an appropriate starting date for your child and possibly even assist you in your efforts.

Think of school as your ally, not as an antagonist. Early childhood programs share in your child's care and education, and are an important partner in your child's early years. If possible, begin a new school relationship with an attitude of mutual decision making and trust.

Sometimes the school experience helps children with the final steps of potty training, as children learn from their pottying peers. For example, the daily routines include potty breaks that often add a predictable structure to potty choices. Lastly, the classroom teacher is often a neutral adult that your child is eager to please.

What is the average age for children to be potty trained?

The answer to this question depends on the definition of potty training. In a Western culture that stresses independence, "potty training" usually includes the entire process from understanding the first need-to-potty sensations to the after-potty self-help skills. A potty trained child feels the need to potty before pottying and is interested in controlling where and when he potties. He can communicate the need to potty and can physically hold it until he gets to a potty. He can remove the necessary clothes to go potty and can wipe himself afterwards.

This complete package called "potty trained" happens somewhere around three years old, with many children needing help wiping bowel movements until they are nearly four years old.

Some children will demonstrate all the potty training skills after their second or third birthday, while others will have a few of the key ingredients, but not all. The potty training process, from the time some of the necessary abilities emerge until the total package "clicks," can take six to eight months. However, this should not be six months of desperation. Rather, it is six months of moving toward self-reliance, while sometimes taking a few steps back.

This learning process leading up to that final finish line might be quick or it might be slow. Just remember, the tortoise and the hare both get to the same goal. However, pushing the tortoise makes him retreat, not go faster.

Is it possible to potty train babies under one year old?

Potty training babies under one year of age is possible. It just means something different than the earlier definition of potty training as an independent skill. Potty training children who are less than one year of age is an interdependent potty venture. The same interdependent philosophy is found in Suzuki music education where the parent learns the instrument before the child so the parent can be a teaching partner.

Mom, or another caregiver, gets the baby to the potty at the right time and assists her in the potty process. This may work better with babies who do well on a schedule. Mom watches the baby for signals that she is ready to go, from grunts to wiggling. Mom carries the baby to the potty, adding a sign or signal of her own; for example, a psssing sound. In time, the baby associates the signal with pottying. Voila, no more diapers!

This process only works with time, attention, and a noncoercive loving partnership. It is not for the overworked and the overscheduled, and not in homes trying to juggle the needs of adults and other family members.

Do girls potty train earlier than boys?

Girls may potty train earlier than boys but, if so, it's only a difference of a few months. Keep in mind that gender differences are statistical differences. They do not predict when your child is ready or when your child will be successful.

Toddler-age girls may have earlier language development. They can then verbalize the potty process and talk about the sequence of events with caregivers. Listening skills also help young children to follow directions better and to think before acting. With earlier language skills, children can communicate their immediate needs and recruit adult help in getting to the closest potty.

Toddler-age boys may be more active at physical play. Energetic boys may master control of their body and limbs but may not be as tuned into the inner workings of their bodies. They may not have the patience to sit for a few minutes on a potty and notice how they can control what comes out.

Timing, of course, is everything. In every case, interest plus developmental landmarks will be the determining factors.

Do boys potty train sitting down or standing up?

If you are the parent of a boy, you have the additional decision of whether to teach your son to pee standing up or sitting down. Usually it's best to keep it simple at first. In the beginning, teach your son to sit to pee and to poop. Once he understands the logistics, he will want to imitate his male role models. When your son is motivated to imitate his stand-up male role models, you can get him a step stool to reach the adult-size toilet.

Same-gender role models can make learning easier. Your child won't need to make any logical inferences about what's the same and what's different if he sees similar anatomy, whether he sees Daddy, older siblings, or male classmates at school. Not to worry, though; there's no evidence that female potty teachers significantly inhibit potty learning.

Are second children easier to potty train?

Siblings are a huge asset to the social aspect of potty training. Little ones learn by example. The more they are immersed in a world of potty-going people, the more they internalize the implicit expectation that this is how it should be done. Then, it's just a matter of time until they discover that their body works the same way.

Older siblings also provide important motivation. Who doesn't want to be just like a respected older brother? Young children are watching the people they love with fearless devotion. That desire will expedite potty learning once the physical control is in place.

But you don't have to go out and borrow an older child during the potty training months. Young children have the uncanny ability to recruit all kinds of interesting people into their potty training world.

Does peer pressure make potty training easier?

Your child's peers become a significant influence on her behavior after three years of age. They often add a new motivation for potty training but only if adults are not adding negative competition to the child's experience. Negative comparisons have a potential for escalating into a power struggle—for example, your child could respond, "Oh yeah…you say look at her. Look at me; I can make your life miserable!" Like natural consequences, let the peer experience do the teaching without emotionally charged lectures comparing children's abilities.

Stick to simple emotionally neutral descriptions when talking about peer behavior. If you invite a potty trained friend to your home during potty play times, let the potty trained child lead the potty experience. Be the "invisible hand" creating opportunities for interest. If your child isn't already curious about her friend's behavior, you won't inspire interest.

Similarly, when your child is at preschool, your prompting may cause resistance. Stand back. Allow your child to observe and choose. Should your child express a desire to "kick the diapers" or show concern that she's the last one wearing diapers, tell her clearly that you are ready to help her. Reintroduce your potty plan.

What is potty training etiquette in public situations?

Once your child is interested in potty training, you might hear him interviewing everyone he sees about their potty preferences—strangers in grocery lines and grandparents included. Everyone in earshot will soon learn what's on your child's learning agenda. Be prepared during the potty training process to discuss seemingly private topics in the most unusual places. That's a good sign you're doing the right thing.

You can begin to teach the nuances of social etiquette by redirecting the conversation. Simply explain to others that your child is excited about potty training. Social graces are best taught by example at this age. Young children do not understand that potty training might not be a proper topic at the holiday dinner table.

Similarly, if your child wants to show others his private body parts, remind him that he should wait until he gets into the bathroom to take off his clothes. Validate his enthusiasm for the new things he is learning and add this to the list of "everything in its place" principle of potty training.

Which comes first—potty training for pee or for poop?

It may seem like potty training for pee comes first since peeing on the potty gets so much of your attention. The real answer to the question depends on your child's physical and emotional readiness.

As your child learns to read the physical sensations of her body, she has more control over where to potty. She may know more clearly that a poop is coming and therefore be more likely to get to the potty in time. Or, she may feel a poop coming and prefer to poop in the diaper because the diaper is more familiar. One child may feel the need to pee, stop everything, and enjoy getting to the potty on time while her twin sister might feel the need to pee, try to hold it until she finishes what she's doing, and rarely make it to the potty in time. Each child is different.

In any case, you should approach potty training the same way in all cases—by teaching the same general principles and creating realistic potty routines. Success will usually come in small steps. Some children will pee on the potty before they poop on the potty. Others will poop on the potty before they pee on the potty. Either way, you will build from your child's initial success.

How do I teach the proper way to wipe after pottying?

Teach your child to wipe from front to back. Shortcuts here turn into poor hygiene habits. Unfortunately, it may take years for your child to perfect thorough wiping. In the long run, wiping away from the vagina will help prevent urinary tract infections.

Since you are your child's first role model, pay attention to how you wipe your child. Be sure to point out that the front to back motion is deliberate, not accidental, as you're doing it. When you start potty practice, as well as anytime you are handling toilet paper, take the opportunity to mention the right way to wipe. Ask your child to show you how she wipes herself. Gently remind her to "clean front to back" and accept all approximations even if you find her "wiping" her tummy instead. That just tells you she still needs your help.

The rest is personal style. Some children may wipe from the back between their legs. Others wipe from in front of their legs. Some are contortionists. Others are dainty. Many different methods work, as long as the job gets done.

Is there anything I should do before my child is ready for potty training?

Yes, you can set a foundation for potty training when your child is a young toddler. Your child does not have a switch that turns on the minute he is ready for potty training. Before you even start potty training, you will change hundreds, maybe thousands, of diapers!

As your child becomes interested in language, use these opportunities to familiarize him with potty language. Explain that you're changing his diaper because it's wet or because there's a poop.

If you notice your child going pee or poop in his diaper, mention it without any expectation to potty train yet. You will be putting words to your child's experience and helping him to understand what his body is doing. This is not a time to joke or laugh at your child, however.

Allow your child to join you in the bathroom. Again, describe what you're doing. You are helping your child to understand the world around him. When you talk about the dog peeing, the cat pooping, or the bird poop on the sidewalk, think of this as a toddler science lesson called "Scientific Observation and Description for Eighteen-Month-Olds." In these ways, you are building a meaningful context for his future potty learning.

What advantages are there to early potty training?

Early potty training has distinct advantages for the parents. The thrill of no more diapers to change is liberating. The financial savings of no more diapers is significant. And then there is the pride that your child has successfully mastered an important childhood landmark. Add an extra "wow" to that pride if your child is the first to be potty trained among her peers.

Does a child, let's say under the age of two, feel additional pride for beating her friends in the potty game? No, young children feel pride in what they can do and don't compare themselves with others at this age. Children feel pride in mastering potty training whenever the time comes that they master potty training.

Children do look to parents and special adults for feedback on their successes. For that reason, you want to be sure that your parenting agenda is consistent with your child's developmental stage. Potty training before your child is ready can increase resistance and delay success. Keep in mind that early potty-goers are not more intelligent than their peers and sustain no long-term advantages.

What advantages are there to late potty training?

The length of the potty training process will be shorter if you wait with patient awareness for your child's readiness signs (see Chapter 2). This will also decrease frustration for you and your child. There is no going forward without the physical ability to stay dry for short periods of time. And you can only inch your child forward without his own personal interest in the goal.

By waiting, you improve the ease of communication. Your child will have the language skills to communicate through the potty training process and the cognitive understanding of what is expected and when.

Some of the obstacles to potty training will be more apparent because your child is an active participant in the potty process. Once he can tell you what's wrong, you will be able to identify appropriate solutions. For example, if he can say "Mommy, it hurts to poop," you know how to change his diet and can help him conquer the physical and emotional discomfort.

Is it possible to wait too long to start potty training?

With all due respect, there is a rare syndrome that affects well-meaning but very tired parents around the time of the third child. It is called Pooped Parent Syndrome. In this situation, the child is ready for potty training and has been for months. However, she is still wearing diapers because it's easier for the parent.

Why might this happen? The parent may want to avoid the mad dash for a public restroom, or be too busy orchestrating all the other aspects of family life. Young children who need to go to the bathroom can be very time consuming.

However, if the child is old enough to ask "Am I wearing diapers or underpants?" in order to make the appropriate choice of whether to potty or not, the child is ready to say good-bye to diapers.

How does potty training affect self-esteem?

Your child's self-esteem is based on a genuine mastery of his world, and in this case of his body. He learns that he is capable of being successful. He also sees his self-worth reflected in the opinions of the people he loves. He feels loved and accepted when he makes mistakes. And he feels supported until he can accomplish an important childhood landmark.

Self-esteem is not founded on empty praise. Your child has an inner sense of what he can and cannot do. Praise is not enough, although positive encouragement is essential. After all, you wouldn't be happy with a cheerleading coworker who praised your work but never shared a critical piece of information that would make your job easier.

Potty training is a partnership with your child, which sets a foundation for your future relationship. You really don't want to miss this incredible bonding opportunity together.

- If your child is struggling because some essential readiness components aren't there, he learns he is not good enough.
- If your child's fears are dismissed as nothing, he learns not to trust his feelings.

- If your child is belittled for accidents, he learns to give up.
- If your child feels too much pressure, he learns to exert control in negative ways.

Is potty training different in different cultures?

Yes, potty training is different in different cultures just as parenting is different in different cultures. Some cultures stress interdependence and cooperation while others stress independence and individualism. However, parenting practices will always be related to your core values about childhood and about learning.

Potty training options are also related to practical factors like economy and local climates. From sanitation systems to infant clothing, everything shapes the way families interact with their babies.

People in many countries around the world, such as African countries, Japan, China, India, and many Latin American countries, potty train babies under one year of age. One way is not better than another. Successful potty training must fit your family's reality.

In a world with so many choices, however, you may feel like you must defend your choice against all others. Or, you have to reach consensus among radically different viewpoints. Your au pair from Venezuela and your mother-in-law from England all want what's best for your child. Your job is to decide what will work in your household at this particular time for this particular child.

Chapter 2

YOUR CHILD IS AN INDIVIDUAL: READINESS AND PERSONALITY

- How do I know when my child is ready for potty training?
- What physical behaviors are important for potty training readiness?
- What emotional behaviors are important for potty training readiness?
- What language behaviors are important for potty training readiness?
- What cognitive behaviors are important for potty training readiness?
- Can I help my child become ready for potty training?
- What are some gentle ways to promote my child's readiness?
- What is a positive potty training environment?
- What situations make potty training more difficult?
- Does a child's temperament affect potty training?
- What are the potty training strengths of an easy temperament?
- What are the potty training challenges of an easy temperament?
- What are the potty training strengths of a difficult temperament?
- What are the potty training challenges of a difficult temperament?
- What are the potty training strengths of a slow-to-warm-up temperament?

- What are the potty training challenges of a slow-to-warm-up temperament?
- Can a child be a combination of temperaments?
- How do I potty train twins or multiple same-age siblings?
- What is my temperament style?
- How does my temperament style affect my potty training success?
- Is potty training at some ages/stages more difficult than in others?
- Is it okay to start and stop the potty training process?
- Do some children show readiness signs between eighteen months and two years old only to stall their progress a few months later?
- If I wait long enough, will my child potty train herself?
- Can a child never be "ready"?

How do I know when my child is ready for potty training?

Usually you see the first signs of potty training readiness on a Monday. It's similar to the early warning tropical weather systems that predict hurricanes a week before landfall. You then have a few days to reread the books, get the proper supplies, phone friends for their helpful advice, and contact family members to clear their schedules for the upcoming potty party. By Friday, you are ready to work with your child and by Sunday, you will be celebrating. NOT!

In potty training, as with all developmental landmarks, there comes a time when you start to wonder, "Is now the time?" Is now the time to feed your baby solid food? Will your baby be crawling soon? Should you begin potty training? Just because you're asking doesn't mean the answer is "Yes, now." However, when you begin asking the readiness question, it is a good time to start observing your child.

Watch and wait for these four areas of readiness: physical development, language development, emotional development, and cognitive development.

- Your child can stay dry for short periods of time.
- Your child can communicate the need to potty before she goes.
- Your child is curious and motivated.
- Your child understands the sequence of before, during, and after, as well as the big picture "This is the way to potty—good-bye diapers."

A list of readiness behaviors follows for each area of development.

What physical behaviors are important for potty training readiness?

Potty training requires your child to understand the inner and outer workings of his body. He begins to understand how his body feels before pottying and make a connection between those feelings and certain actions. He learns that a full bladder makes him pee and pressure on his bottom makes a poop.

Usually if children are busy mastering other physical milestones, they are not ready to move forward to a new one like potty training. Running and climbing usually precede pottying because they bring your child pure joy in and of themselves. Give your child time to enjoy physical movement before asking him to use those movements to meet other goals.

The physical behaviors:

- Your child stays dry for at least two hours during the day.
- Your child wakes up dry from naps.
- Your child will pee or poop regularly—before bath time, or an hour after breakfast.
- You see telltale signs when your child is pottying—he stops playing, makes a certain face, or squats in a more private part of the room.
- Your child can walk to a designated place to accomplish a goal.
- Your child can remove pieces of clothing to use the potty.

What emotional behaviors are important for potty training readiness?

All learning for young children involves an emotional component. Your child makes a personal connection to every new skill: "This is fun.".... "This makes me happy.".... "I want to do this again!" This component is especially important, because potty training involves some risks—age-appropriate risks, but risks just the same.

During potty training, your child may face disappointment, confusion, mistakes, and fears. Temperament, timing, environment, and routines are all precedents for how your child learns to handle age-appropriate dilemmas. If your child is intrigued by the potty process, the thrill of mastery will overshadow the obstacles along the way.

The emotional behaviors:

- Your child asks questions about pottying.
- Your child wants to follow others into the bathroom.
- Your child tries to imitate adult potty behavior.
- Your child likes clean diapers—she asks to be changed at appropriate times.
- Your child cares about the outcomes of her actions—she expresses likes or dislikes after

she does something and if reminded will remember those preferences the next time.

- Your child is willing to sit still to master a task.

What language behaviors are important for potty training readiness?

Language changes your child's world. With language, your child organizes ideas into a sequence of before, during, and after. Your child talks about past events— for example, what happened last time he sat on the potty. He also makes predictions about "What happens if . . . ?" such as, "If I ask for help, someone helps me."

Through language, your child takes control of his world. He describes needs and wants. He asks for help. Language also opens the door for imagination. Your child can now replay situations again and again in his play as he internalizes new skills.

The verbal behaviors:

- Your child knows his body parts.
- Your child can tell you, first when he's pottied in his diaper, and then before he's pottied in his diaper.
- Your child follows simple directions— "Quick, run to the bathroom!"
- Your child tells you what he needs.
- Your child says he wants to "do it myself."

What cognitive behaviors are important for potty training readiness?

Language leads to more elaborate thinking. Your child makes plans. She coordinates actions and people to accomplish her goals. Actions have a purpose and the world responds to the things she does. She knows she can be cute and capable and plans her actions accordingly.

Unless your child is chasing a bright red ball into the street, your child begins to think and act at the same time. She is aware that she is an active participant in the potty training experience. She now chooses actions that reflect her motivations.

The cognitive behaviors:

- Your child is curious about how her body works.
- Your child sees the connection between her body and the potty.
- Your child understands sequencing— before, during, and after.
- Your child lines up her toys—understands order—things in "right" places.
- Your child thinks ahead—she can stop doing something if she needs to potty.
- Your child comprehends that potty books and videos are relevant to her actions at this time.

• Your child understands the "big picture"—
"So, this is how things work?"

Can I help my child become ready for potty training?

Sometimes attention to the readiness factors opens the door to a new stage. When you wondered about your child crawling, you started putting toys just a little farther from his reach. This encouraged your child to try new movements. Your attention encouraged your child to do something new and exciting. At the same time, you were careful not to frustrate your baby.

Anything you do to support your child's development is about making discoveries with your child. This is not an urgent intervention—you are not doing something "to" your child. Instead, use a gentle curiosity to explore what your child knows and what your child wants.

Before embarking on a potty agenda, you should consider the type of preliminary information you are giving your child. Have you talked about potty behavior in general? Do you make bathroom routines as interesting as story times? After all, learning about bodies and bathrooms is certainly appealing to children.

While you can immerse your child in the natural experience of pottying, you cannot change when your child will acquire the physical control of actually peeing and pooping. That's one area of readiness where you have to sit back and wait.

What are some gentle ways to promote my child's readiness?

Your child may be ready in one area of potty skills but not in all potty areas. Use these gentle strategies to create a more balanced potty readiness profile. Start by noticing connections between your child's behavior and the area of her strength. Build new opportunities for connections in the areas that are lacking.

You can promote physical readiness by recognizing when your child takes charge of her body. Notice when your child pees or poops in her diaper and tell her that's what she's doing. You will be adding to her awareness of what her body does.

You can promote emotional readiness by including your child in your bathroom routine. Again, this is as natural as having your child watch you talk on the phone and then imitate your behavior.

You can promote language readiness by adding language to daily potty activities. Talk about what you're doing and ask your child engaging questions. Talking about pottying is just like asking your child to point to the moon or identify the color of grass—it is just ordinary day-to-day interaction.

Similarly, talking to your child about pottying may create a new cognitive awareness. You may be holding the missing link that your child is looking for. Start with neutral descriptions of your behavior— "Wait here while mommy goes to the potty. I drank a lot of water today."

In every instance, however, give up the explanations if your child looks bored. Wait for a better time when your child will give you positive feedback.

What is a positive potty training environment?

Your child picks up multiple cues from his environment. These inconspicuous messages can support or hinder your attempts at potty training. A positive atmosphere is a must. You want potty training time to be geared to your child's body, your child's way of thinking, and your child's needs.

- Potty training should be fun, as your child learns through play. Giggles always improve your chances of success.
- Potty gear should be helpful rather than overly complicated. For example, batteries

are probably not necessary for potty equipment. The right size and the right fit will give your child all the security he needs.

- Bathrooms should be child-friendly. Your child does not want to spend time in a place he's told is dirty and disgusting.
- Routines should be stable and predictable. Your child is learning to pay attention to significant moments in his day. You can make that easier if your child can guess when those moments are most likely to happen.
- Schedules should be relaxed. Eliminate the frantic need to be in too many places at once. If you do, your child will have time to think.
- Expectations should be opportunities for success. Unrealistic demands and the threat of failure undermine the process of learning from mistakes.
- Choose easy-to-clean clothes and surfaces. Fancy clothes and new carpeting add to your frustration without adding anything to your child's learning.

What situations make potty training more difficult?

If simplicity works in your favor, life's complications work against your child's success. Changes can unsettle your child. However, keep in mind that your child experiences her world up-close and personal. For example, travel might throw off her sleep schedule, but having her favorite teddy bear and hearing her special lullaby can make everything just right.

The following situations may complicate your child's potty training experience. See Chapter 3 for strategies to make the best of these situations.

- A new baby in the house takes time-consuming support away from your child's potty efforts and also presents the confusing suggestion that babies get all the attention.
- Changing your child's sleep routine from the crib to a bed requires another dimension of independence if your child is already on shaky ground.
- Traveling may disrupt well-established schedules and routines.
- Moving to a new house changes the routines and the familiarity of the environment.

- Any changes that draw energy and effort away from your child will impact potty training: new jobs, new schools, family stresses.

Does a child's temperament affect potty training?

Your child was born with a temperament style that was evident within the first twenty-four hours and that will be there when he goes to off to college. After all, your personal temperament style that was on full display as a child is still in you today as a parent. Luckily, you have had many years to learn to compensate for times when your temperament makes situations more challenging.

Temperament affects how you learn and how you handle change. It also affects potty training.

Nearly four decades ago, two researchers, Chess and Thomas, professors of child psychiatry and psychiatry, respectively, identified three different temperament styles: easy, slow-to-warm-up, and difficult. According to their now-classic research, Chess and Thomas found these three temperament styles reflect differences in the nine characteristics listed below.

1. Activity level
2. Regularity
3. Distractibility
4. Intensity

5. Sensitivity
6. Adaptability
7. Persistence
8. Approach/Withdrawal
9. Mood

Each temperament style has strengths and weaknesses. The "easy child" may be flexible and open to new situations but may not tell you forcefully if he experiences physical discomfort. The "easy" child is not happier than the other temperaments, but won't create a scene over "nothing." The "difficult child" does not have an intrinsic flaw. He just gets stuck because he can doggedly pursue his agenda and protests forcefully if you don't understand. The "slow-to-warm-up child" always takes his time to observe and grow into new situations.

What are the potty training strengths of an easy temperament?

The child with an easy temperament is the easiest to potty train.

1. She is less frenetic and able to sit for short lengths of time.

2. She adapts well to schedules. Feeding schedules and nap schedules are predictable, which also leads to a predictable potting schedule.

3. She isn't easily distracted from a task. So, if she sees a new toy on her way to the bathroom, she will remember to come back to it after she goes potty.

4. She can listen to verbal encouragement and support without a strong emotional reaction.

5. The sensory experience of sitting on a cold potty or of a naked bottom is not overwhelming.

6. She will respond easily to pottying in a variety of situations under a variety of conditions. She is more likely to pause one activity if she needs to take a potty break.

7. Her frustration may be expressed more mildly. Mistakes and setbacks will be small blips to success rather than major pitfalls.

8. She may be eager to embrace new potty expectations. For example, she may be eager to sit on a new potty. She may even claim to be ready before physical readiness is apparent.

9. Overall, the potty process is more likely to be light-hearted. You may experience quick success or steady progress instead of an emotional roller coaster.

What are the potty training challenges of an easy temperament?

The child with an easy temperament may not care if he needs a clean diaper. He is not distressed by the minor inconveniences of diapers. The motto "life is good" was written for him.

The child with an easy temperament may not ask to be potty trained. If you ask him to use a potty, he will. But if you don't ask him, he's equally content. And if you're a busy parent, you might be relieved that he doesn't seem to need you. This is also the child who doesn't set off loud alarms when she has an ear infection and probably won't complain about urinary tract infections or painful stools, either. This child could be the last to be potty trained, simply from benign neglect. In this case, if you hear your inner voice asking "Hmmmm, I wonder if he's ready?" it may be time to take a few simple steps that move your child forward into the next stage. You may be happily surprised at the easy results.

What are the potty training strengths of a difficult temperament?

The child with a difficult temperament probably won't potty train without some concentrated effort. This child likes things "her way" but will respond to clear expectations and attentive support.

1. Potty training is a physical activity. This child may not love sitting still but she may love running to

the potty or pulling the toilet paper when she's finished. You can give timely reminders to keep your child's activity level focused—"First potty, then we'll pull this much toilet paper…and STOP." Teaching "stop" is a game, not a threat.

2. The child with a difficult temperament can be unpredictable in her schedule. This is a strength if you are a flexible parent. You will naturally check in on your child's needs rather than expect today to resemble yesterday.

3. All children believe adult attention is the raison d'etre, especially the child with the difficult temperament. Your genuine engagement outweighs any other distraction and will be a powerful resource while potty training a child with a difficult temperament.

4. The child with a difficult temperament likes to do things in "a big way." Use this trait to create big potty training excitement.

5. The child with a difficult temperament will experience every nuance of the potty training experience. If you tune in to her sensory world, you can make the necessary adjustments and give her explicit verbal descriptions of her feelings.

6. The child with a difficult temperament likes to feel in control. You can turn this into a positive by

letting her feel like she's choosing where, when, and how to potty. Of course, you must remain the invisible hand orchestrating her success.

7. The child with a difficult temperament hates to give up. Use this as a potty training strength by focusing on the small successes that bring your child closer to ultimate success.

8. The child with a difficult temperament will vehemently protest change. You can honor this child's voice—say it loud and say it strong—without you, the parent, collapsing in self-doubt.

9. This child may say "NO!" when she really means "maybe." She also wants to wear underpants one day. The world is full of high maintenance people—artists, scientists, inventors. You will have great stories to tell and possibly develop a great sense of humor along the way.

What are the potty training challenges of a difficult temperament?

The child with a difficult temperament will be the most challenging to potty train. But remember, this is not about you as the parent doing things wrong and it's not about the child deliberately making your life stressful. This is the way your child approaches new situations. This is how he was born.

You cannot change a child's temperament. You can, however, teach your child to make the most of his strengths. He can learn how he will respond in different situations and will eventually learn successful strategies to compensate for challenging moments.

This requires time and energy on your part, especially during the potty training years. Your child needs you to help regulate his experiences until he learns self-control. He is stuck wanting control and hating change—stuck between too much and too little. It's up to you to build the bridge that will take him across.

Because the child with the difficult temperament resists change, he may not feel "ready" for potty training. You will have to observe readiness characteristics on your own and start building that bridge. You may have to work hard to win his "buy-in." But once you have it, he won't let anything stand in his way.

What are the potty training strengths of a slow-to-warm-up temperament?

The child with a slow-to-warm-up temperament can appear easy because of her quiet nature. She handles change well when it is introduced slowly, allowing her to gradually become comfortable and confident in new situations.

1. The child with a slow-to-warm-up temperament is often described as watchful. She likes to be prepared before taking action. This is a strong positive for potty training because she is the least impulsive of the three temperament styles.

2. This child's mild disposition complements the predictability of a potty training routine. She likes to know what's happening next.

3. The child with a slow-to-warm-up temperament is the classic tortoise moving steadfastly toward a goal. It may take her longer, but she always gets there.

4. You won't have loud power struggles with a child who has a slow-to-warm-up temperament. Your child voices opposition in less direct ways.

5. The child with a slow-to-warm-up temperament may seem very sensitive to the physical sensations of potty training. You can give her orienting cues of new sensations to ease her hesitancy. For example, she will think it's a game if you remind her to listen to the pee falling in the toilet.

6. The slow-to-warm-up child likes learning new skills. She just needs to do it on her own time schedule. With adequate preparation, she does adapt.

7. The slow-to-warm-up child can accomplish anything in the world. She just may need a hand to hold along the way.

8. This child definitely tends to linger on the sidelines rather than jump forward with both feet (until you really get to know her, that is). The good news is you probably won't find her upturning potty chairs and running wildly through the park without her pants.

9. Her mood is cautious more than negative or positive. This will give you time to adjust your potty training to fit her needs.

What are the potty training challenges of a slow-to-warm-up temperament?

Potty training a child with a slow-to-warm-up temperament can be exhausting if you don't want to revisit each step each and every day. This child loves repetition to a fault. So, prepare yourself to work more closely with his timetable.

Because the child with a slow-to-warm-up temperament has a tendency to withdraw in new situations, he may withdraw instead of asking for help when he needs it. Don't jump in and rescue him. Simply remind him you are there to help if he asks.

The child with the slow-to-warm-up temperament tends to register his unhappiness mildly. Therefore, he could get a little whiney. Let him know you are happy to help but he needs to ask for help in appropriate ways. Similarly, watch out for quiet subversion. In his attempt to buy more time, he can sabotage his own success.

The biggest obstacle to potty training a child with a slow-to-warm-up temperament occurs if you are an action-oriented parent. There will be days when you want to strangle your child. Don't get frustrated— this child cannot be rushed.

Can a child be a combination of temperaments?

Parents usually see aspects of different temperament styles in each individual child. And, of course, your child didn't read the research. The important message behind the research on temperament styles is that the adults must modify their interactions to complement the child's strengths.

Some combinations of temperament styles often sound counterintuitive. For example, your child might be easy and difficult at the same time. She might enjoy new people and places, and be the first to join a group. Yet when she falls apart, she does so with shocking fury. This happens consistently, whether she is an infant or in her "terrible two's."

Or, your child might be slow-to-warm-up and difficult. She could be the happiest kid on the block at home where the routine is consistent and predictable. But when faced with a new situation, she may need slow, frequent repetition. And if she gets frustrated, she loses the ability to stand back and regroup. Instead she shouts an earth shattering "NO!" and runs to the farthest reaches of the house.

The best potty training practices will work for most children most of the time. You will also carry a little bag of parenting tricks that adapts to your child's unique personality.

How do I potty train twins or multiple same-age siblings?

Even though children are born at the same time from the same parents, it does not mean they will have the same potty training schedule. Each child has a unique temperament style and his or her own personal developmental clock. You may have one child who is a potty natural, leading the way to easy, early success. Your other child may not be interested until months later. And when she is ready, her potty training style may be completely different than that of her sibling.

It is best not to assume both children will complete potty training at the exact same time. Try to form your expectations for each individual child by looking at his or her readiness traits separately. Create the same positive potty environment for both children but plan on modifying your potty plan to meet each child's individual needs. One child may want to do everything by herself while the other wants your hands-on support. One might strongly dislike diapers while the other relishes the security.

However, there are advantages to potty training same-age siblings together. For example, they can learn from watching one another. A hesitant child sees the confidence of a bold child. A child who doesn't comprehend pieces in the potty process has her best friend there to show her. They help each other. They laugh together. They grow together. Enjoy potty training as a team, but remember everyone on the team has different strengths.

What is my temperament style?

Temperament styles are still very much part of your adult personality. You have learned many adaptive strategies to camouflage less effective temperament traits, but those traits are just under the surface and show up when you least expect. Your genuine temperament style comes out when you are most yourself with close friends and family.

Are you mostly an easygoing, adaptable, flexible, go-with-the-flow person? Would people describe you as even-tempered without a lot of peaks and valleys? When things go wrong, do you respond mildly and easily move on to the next thing?

Or, do you like to be well-prepared in new situations—do you rehearse speeches and practice skills many times in advance? Does it take others a little time to get to know the real you? Do you plan ahead what to wear to a new place and practice a few tried-and-true conversation starters or jokes to break the ice?

Or, do you like things "your way" and "now"? Would others describe you as meticulous or intense? A great description of an adult with a difficult temperament is Meg Ryan's character in the movie When Harry Met Sally. This woman likes her salad dressing on the side and the pie a la mode heated with strawberry ice cream, not vanilla…no, change that…make it whipped cream instead of ice cream but only if it's real whipped cream! Sound familiar? People with "high maintenance" temperaments are everywhere and we love 'em!

How does my temperament style affect my potty training success?

You want your expectations to match your child's temperament style. Otherwise, you're headed for a highly stressful potty training experience. If you and your child share a temperament style, you will intu-itively know what to expect from your child. You will also already have an abundance of adaptive strategies to help your child be successful.

There is also the possibility that you wish your child did not have your temperament style. You may wish he were more assertive than cautious like you. Or, you may wish he would just let a problem go instead of dwelling on it for hours. Self-acceptance will serve you well here. You can also recruit potty partners who do not take your child's behaviors personally.

If you and your child have different temperament styles, you might approach your child with unrealis-tic assumptions. The parent with an easy tempera-ment might grow exhausted by a child with a difficult temperament—it's not easy. The parent with a difficult temperament might approach potty train-ing with more intensity than is warranted. The parent with a slow-to-warm-up temperament might still be thoroughly researching potty training long after the child is ready. You are who you are. Parenting gives you that incredible opportunity to learn about your-self as you learn about your child.

Is potty training at some ages/stages more difficult than in others?

Potty training is more complicated when your child is in one of those oppositional stages. Oppositional stages can intensify counterproductive power struggles between you and your child, adding stress and delays to the potty process.

The first of these oppositional stages occurs when your child is around eighteen months of age, or the first time she says "No" and "Mine." In this stage, she is pushing away from you to become her own person. Every "no" challenges the world to acknowledge her. She feels powerful and likes the way it feels. "Mine" is her way of defining herself and her place in the world. She rules the world by making a claim on everything she touches.

Somewhere around two-and-a-half years old, you will witness another highly volatile stage. Your child will be experiencing a new set of highly charged emotions to complement new gains in language development. Your emerging little person is now confronted by fears, frustration, anger, and jealousy.

These stages trump all other learning because your child's emotional growth requires front and center status. Growth spurts usually create a temporary but necessary imbalance. Wait a few months for potty training and your cooperative child will return, ready to tackle new challenges with a renewed sense of strength.

Is it okay to start and stop the potty training process?

You begin potty training with optimism. While you may plan on a few minor detours along the way, you should not plan on stopping once you begin. It is better to invest in thorough planning, wait for readiness, and believe you can win your child's cooperation before committing to regular potty visits.

Your child has more likelihood for success if surrounded by clear, consistent potty messages. Throwing up your hands in frustration while saying, "I quit. This isn't worth it!" is not an option. Calmly saying to your child, "I don't want to fight about pottying. We'll try again another time" is acceptable. The first gives your child mixed messages. The second is a mutually acceptable time-out.

The difference may sound like semantics to you, but not to your child. Words create your child's reality. Never give up. The ultimate goal is always in focus—it is just a little farther away than you first imagined. So, take a step back if your child is increasingly negative, defiant, or averse to the potty training.

Shift your effort to address those feelings before continuing with a potty training agenda.

Stopping is like getting a "get out of jail free" card. You may need it, but use it wisely.

Do some children show readiness signs between eighteen months and two years old only to stall their progress a few months later?

Your child between eighteen months and two years old may demonstrate an interest and an ability in potty training, particularly if he is not in an intense "No" stage. This is a time of enormous growth and development as monumental as the transition into the teen years. You may also be an inspiring cheerleader who is ready to take him to the potty every few hours.

If you are both enjoying the time and the attention, this may lead to long-term success. However, it doesn't always. Often, the novelty of the experience wears off for one or both of you. Your child may not be ready to assume more responsibility for the potty experience for six to eight more months.

- Does your child really feel the sensation of needing to go to the potty without your reminders?

- Is he willing to initiate a request for help if you forget to ask him?
- Does he really care about potty training or does he love potty training with you?

Stay with it if you're okay continuing this hands-on approach for an indefinite amount of time. Consider that there will be other preliminary strategies you can use at this time without potty training defining the majority of your interactions with your child.

If I wait long enough, will my child potty train herself?

A small number of children do seem to potty train themselves. They wake up one day ready to use a potty and never look back to diapers again. They are most likely children with an easy temperament. If this happens, you should go buy a lottery ticket to parlay your good fortune. In other words, it happens, but not often.

Most children do not potty train themselves. Instead, your child welcomes guidance and support from you. Even with all the readiness factors in place, you still have a job to do:

- You describe.
- You explain.
- You answer questions, spoken and unspoken.

- You teach problem solving.
- You have the ability to abstract information to new contexts and explain again.
- You teach how to handle change, setbacks, and mistakes.
- You become a measure of successes, large and small.
- You give love and make everything worthwhile.

Why are you waiting? You're waiting for readiness, not for your child to do it herself.

Can a child never be "ready"?

Typically developing children will all be ready for potty training one day. If it seems like your child is not anywhere near his peers in potty training, look at how he's doing in the areas of development: motor skills, language skills, cognitive skills, social skills, self-control, and emotional literacy. Potty training is one small part of overall development.

Your child may just not be ready when you're ready. In one possible scenario, your child may have a slow-to-warm-up temperament style that is cautious to the point of not being able to take that necessary step forward. Sometimes, you can give your child a gentle push to experience his long-awaited success.

Alternatively, you may be the person who isn't ready. By the time your child is three years old, you should be involved in some sort of supportive potty training. At a minimum, you will be creating a positive potty environment and establishing the foundation for future readiness.

Chapter 3

CUSTOM-MADE STRATEGIES FOR YOUR FAMILY

- How and when do I prepare for potty training?
- What's the next step when my child shows an interest in potty training?
- What is the most basic potty training strategy?
- What's the "Happy Potty" song?
- Will the basic plan work for all parents?
- How can the basic plan be adapted for "unstructured" parents?
- How can the basic plan be adapted for "weekend warrior" parents?
- How can the basic plan be adapted for busy parents?
- How can the basic plan be adapted for "full house" parents?
- How can the basic plan be adapted into afternoon mini-sessions?
- How can the basic plan be adapted into weekend mini-sessions?
- Does potty training on "Naked Noons" and "Weekend Mini's" take longer than the "Potty Weekend"?
- Are the consecutive days of "Naked Noons" better than the two-days-on/five-days-off of weekend "Potty Play Days"?
- How can the basic plan be adapted for a child with a slow-to-warm-up temperament?
- How can the basic plan be adapted for a child with a difficult temperament?

- Can I teach my child to poop on the potty before teaching to pee on the potty?
- Should I give my child a diaper to poop in if requested?
- Should I call potty training a "big boy" or "big girl" behavior?
- What is the best time to start potty training if I am pregnant or getting ready to adopt another baby?
- Should I start potty training if I am moving into a new home?
- Should I wait to move my child from a crib to a bed during potty training?
- Is it better to wait to begin potty training if we are planning to travel?
- How can I make potty training easier when traveling?
- What can I do when I feel guilty that potty training coincides with seemingly negative events?

How and when do I prepare for potty training?

You prepare for potty training when your child is between eighteen months and two years old. At this time of potty preparation, do not expect anything from your child. You are building the stage and adding some of the scenery. You haven't written the script yet and you're probably months away from rehearsals.

- Establish a positive potty training attitude.
- Choose your potty words.
- Include your child in your bathroom routines.
- Make friends with a potty chair.

- Talk about your child's diapers and potty routines.
- Add a few potty books to your child's home library.
- Begin to interview friends and colleagues, if desired.
- Casually observe children six to twelve months older than your child, if desired.

Use this time to think about your child's temperament style. Watch your child's reaction to the new stimulus you are presenting. This is a stage for your child's future success—make it appealing for him.

What's the next step when my child shows an interest in potty training?

The signs suggest your child is ready. She is initiating potty behavior: She wants to sit on her potty. She doesn't like wearing diapers. She likes the idea of doing things the way Mommy does them.

Follow your child's lead. Add a few potty routines to her daily schedule—have her sit on the potty chair after a nap if she has a dry diaper and after undressing before bath time. Make simple connections between your child's behavior and the potty.

Do not assume at this point that she's ready to run the potty marathon, as she has no idea what the potty marathon is yet. Start explaining the "big picture"—that when she's a little older, she won't wear diapers anymore. Watch and listen. Is she as comfortable saying good-bye to diapers as she is ready to say hello to pink princess underpants?

Now is the time to reread the readiness behavior lists in Chapter 2. This is a time of exploration for your child and a time for you to evaluate how quickly or slowly to advance to the next level.

What is the most basic potty training strategy?

At some point, your child will advance from casual, some-of-the-time potty experiences to that new goal of using a potty instead of a diaper. Your child may wake up one day and say, "No more diapers." Or, the timing might be just right—for example, you may have a ready child and a long weekend with no other obligations in which to give it a try.

- Name the event. A name reinforces the message you're trying to convey to your child—"Hooray, it's a 'Potty Weekend'!"
- Tell your child the goal—"We'll play and potty at home all weekend. Then you can say bye-bye to your diapers."
- Practice the goal under the simplest conditions.

Your plan for the weekend is all about making pottying simple and easy for your child. Take off the diapers so your child can feel his body working. Dress him in easy-off clothing or no clothes at all. He will then have immediate feedback as to what happens without a diaper and an easier time getting on the potty in a timely way.

- Teach potty hygiene. Bathrooms are very fun places without obvious boundaries. Start with clear messages about how to use the toilet paper, how many times to flush the toilet, and a fun hand-washing habit. Sing the "Happy Potty" song to teach children how long hand washing should take.

- Practice makes perfect. Athletes and musicians know repetition is essential to mastery. The beauty of a concentrated "Potty Weekend" is that you are creating the opportunity for repeated success. You are the time management expert for the weekend. It's up to you to take your child for potty breaks every two hours. Focus on the adventure of discovery and the satisfaction of success— "Look, you peed on the potty!"

- A happy ending. No matter what happens on this weekend, you've hopefully had a very personal, fun-filled time with your child. Tell your child how much you enjoyed being with him. If your child is ready, gift wrap those favorite underpants. If your child is still learning, focus on the successes rather than the failures. You aren't finished yet, so read about "Weekend Mini's" for Sunday night potty celebrations. Either way, you have everything you need to evaluate your child's future potty training behavior.

What's the "Happy Potty" song?
Happy potty to me.
Happy potty to me.
I'm learning where to pee.
Happy potty to me!
Happy potty to me.
Happy potty to me.
I'm learning where to poopie.
Happy potty to me!

Will the basic plan work for all parents?

You must adapt the basic plan to you and your family according to your temperament or your lifestyle. Parents with a more laid back temperament may rebel against the structure of a "Potty Weekend." Highly structured parents may lose the personal connection with their child because they get lost in the rigidity of the rules. Some adults may get bored staying home all weekend. Busy multitasking pros may overestimate how many other things they can include in the "Potty Weekend." Some may never find a weekend to turn off the outside world. Families with multiple siblings may have too many obligations to devote one weekend to a single child.

That's life. Since parenting is never done in a vacuum, all effective strategies must be modified to fit your very real current situation.

How can the basic plan be adapted for "unstructured" parents?

Unstructured parents may feel too confined by a "Potty Weekend." You will sabotage the consistent routine and hence fail to give clear expectations and support. If you're an unstructured parent, you should:

> • Solicit the help of someone who can keep you on-task; for example a phone-a-friend

who will call every few hours throughout the weekend.

- Recruit another family member to be a hands-on substitute or teaching partner.
- Try regular mini-sessions; for example "naked" afternoons when you can commit to a few hours of a simplified potty routine.

How can the basic plan be adapted for "weekend warrior" parents?

Weekend warriors may be too intense for a "Potty Weekend." They have a tendency to overwhelm the child who did not receive a soft immersion in the potty plan all week long. Weekend warriors should:

- Double-check their preliminary efforts the two weeks preceding the "Potty Weekend." Remember, potty training is a long distance marathon that requires warm-up time, not a cold sprint.
- Relax. Begin the "Potty Weekend" and each individual day with a calming affirmation— "I teach with love and kindness."
- Include preplanned fun activities to balance the tendency to be consumed by a potty agenda. Open-ended activities—blocks,

trucks, new dancing songs, and games—
work best for long days at home.

How can the basic plan be adapted for busy parents?

Life is busy. There are times in your life when you
must juggle more than a sane number of balls in the
air. The potty training months may coincide with a
critical project at work. Your mother-in-law could be
recuperating in your house from a hospital proce-
dure. You try to "do it all" with grace and optimism.
Here are some modifications that may help different
personality types:

- Working parents integrate mini-sessions
  with other child care routines.
- Overdoers solicit a realistic time management buddy to review their plans before
  they begin their "Potty Weekend."
- "Yes" people inform friends and family that
  they are in retreat to minimize tempting
  distractions.
- Perfectionists accept that there will never
  be a perfect time and do it anyway.
- In all cases, parents can substitute the afternoon mini-sessions or try multiple weekend
  mini-sessions.

How can the basic plan be adapted for "full house" parents?

You may have too many other family obligations to devote one weekend to a single child. Older siblings have karate and ballet on opposite sides of town. You're coaching the Sunday afternoon game. Don't forget the pancake breakfast and religious services. Full-house families must either use advance planning or substitute more realistic mini-alternatives.

- Give everyone in the family a part in the potty plan. Create a potty training team with designated "fun" assignments for older and even younger siblings.
- Preplan. Send siblings to sleep-aways at friends or relatives.
- Consider the afternoon mini-sessions or try multiple weekend mini-sessions.

How can the basic plan be adapted into afternoon mini-sessions?

Your goal is to distinguish this particular afternoon as a special time to practice new behaviors. Just like the "Potty Weekend," it also reminds you not to schedule too many other things. By taking these steps, you are 100 percent available to support your child's skill building. At the same time, your child perceives this time as fun and casual with you as the attention-giving bonus.

- Name the time. Since "Naked Noons" is fun to say, it must also be fun to do. Your new "Naked Noons" are meaningful part of a daily routine just like daily story-time.

- Tell your child the goal. "'Naked Noons' is our time everyday to play and potty at home. Then you can say bye-bye to your diapers."

- Practice the goal under the simplest conditions. Begin "Naked Noon" with a ritual starting time. Ring the timer. Sing a song. Now it's time to take off your child's clothes or change out of her diaper into pull-ups. For the next three to four hours, you will be busy playing and doing simple chores while always waiting and watching for potty opportunities. Given that your child is already staying dry longer, your potty breaks will be every hour or hour and a half.

- Teach potty hygiene. Even when potty attempts are futile, you are still reinforcing great bathroom behavior, such as using "just enough" toilet paper, the proper way to wipe, fearless flushing, and of course washing hands to the "Happy Potty" song.

- Practice makes perfect. Schedule "Naked Noons" for two weeks. It's better to include weekend afternoons in your plan, if possible. If not, assume you may need a third week. You will have a good idea of your child's improvement over that period of time and how much longer, if any, you need to proceed.
- A happy ending. You don't want to be held hostage to your "Naked Noons." Their effectiveness ends when you or your child is wishing to be anywhere else but here. Plan for a realistic "happy ending." At the end of the first week, plan to acknowledge some achievement by your child. You may not be shopping for underpants if your child isn't ready, but you can buy some new fun hand towels or character soaps, or make a photo book with pictures from the week called "My Naked Noons."

How can the basic plan be adapted into weekend mini-sessions?

In some households, you cannot commit to two or three consecutive days of potty training, and your weekday schedules do not allow for consistent afternoon sessions. If that's the case, you can plan one month of mini-sessions on Saturdays and Sundays, two to three hours in the morning or in the afternoon. Pick the time of day that matches your child's best mood. If your child hits the day running, choose mornings. If your child sleeps late and hits his stride after lunch, choose afternoons.

- Name the time. You can stick with "Naked Noons" or try "Potty Play Days."

- Tell your child the goal. "This weekend we'll have 'Potty Play Days' to play and potty at home. Then, in a few weeks, you can say bye-bye to your diapers."

- Practice the goal under the simplest conditions. Start your "Potty Play Time" just like "Naked Noons," with a ritual starting time. Now it's time to take off your child's clothes or change him out of his diaper into pull-ups. Plan your "weekend mini-sessions" realistically. Designate a time span that will give your child adequate practice. You will want to "watch and wait" for at least two to three potty opportunities each "Potty Play Day."

- Teach potty hygiene. Continue with fun bathroom rituals—using "just enough" toilet paper, the proper way to wipe, fearless flushing, and of course washing hands to the "Happy Potty" song. Your child is learning through repetition. Each happy bathroom-time reinforces a positive goal.

- Practice makes perfect. Schedule "Potty Play Days" for four consecutive weekends. Because there are five off days in between your "Potty Play Days," you may need additional weekends. The purpose of these "Potty Play Days" is to create successful experiences for your child. Do not continue, however, if your child is not making the connection between taking off his diapers and the choice to pee on the potty. However, if your child asks, allow him to go without diapers during the week in controlled settings.

- A happy ending. "Potty Play Days" are supposed to be a fun time spent together. At the end of each weekend, plan to acknowledge your child's achievement. Were you counting all the times he peed and pooped on the toilet? After Sunday night dinner, present a "Happy Potty" cake with candles for each time your child used the potty. Save the burnt candles. The cake will shine brighter and brighter each week and you can have fun counting all the candles at the end of the month.

Does potty training on "Naked Noons" and "Weekend Mini's" take longer than the "Potty Weekend"?

"Naked Noons" and "Weekend Mini's" do take longer because you are spreading the routine out over a longer period of time. However, they may not necessarily take more total hours. All three strategies lead to the same happy place. Keep in mind that your child, more than any other factor, sets the timing on reaching that ultimate potty training goal.

Quicker is not always better. If "Potty Weekend" is not right for your child or for your family, whether it's because of logistics or temperament, you'll be facing "Sad Sunday," not "Successful Sunday."

Choose your pace honestly and realistically given the best information you have today. Your choice tells you how to pace your efforts. The sprinter is not a better athlete than the marathoner. They are simply running different races. Nonetheless, both are winners.

Are the consecutive days of "Naked Noons" better than the two-days-on/five-days-off of weekend "Potty Play Days"?

Yes, children adapt quicker to a consistent routine but, as mentioned, the actual speed of potty training is irrelevant. What matters is your child's intellectual and emotional ability to participate in "Potty Play Days." Just as your child learns that some of the rules at Grandma's house are different from some of the rules at Mommy's house, she can learn that days without diapers are fun and different. "Potty Play Days" work because your child is ready to learn a new potty routine. She will eventually tell you she's ready and be able to throw away the weekday diapers.

You can still build continuity with your child's weekday routine, particularly if your child is in a child care setting during the week. Talk about similarities and differences to the weekday routines. Send pictures of your child's "Potty Play Days" to your child's teacher. Celebrate school successes at home and celebrate home successes at school.

How can the basic plan be adapted for a child with a slow-to-warm-up temperament?

Children with a slow-to-warm-up temperament need time to adapt to change. You can give your slow-to-warm-up child time in a few different ways:

- Extend the length of potty preparation time. Your slow-to-warm-up child wants to practice his potty skills a little at a time and over a long period of time. He prefers mastery in small manageable pieces rather than in big bites. Stretch his competence slowly by adding new skills and new challenges.

- Use the "Potty Weekend" as the culmination of months of increasingly successful potty behavior. The slow-to-warm-up child does not like surprises. Hold off on the "Potty Weekend" until you are confident that mastery is already there for your child. The weekend then is more of a ritual farewell to diapers than a teaching time.

- "Naked Noons" give a slow-to-warm-up child the opportunity for gradual success with an involved supportive parent. The slow-to-warm-up child also likes the extended daily routine. Anchor the new routine to simple reassuring messages. For example, "When I go on the potty, I don't need my diaper—hip hip hooray for me!" Before you know it, you will hear your child repeat those same words to himself as he moves forward through the potty process.

• Weekend "Potty Play Days" are a second option leading to gradual success. The gap in between practice days is manageable for children with strong verbal and cognitive development because they can talk about "what's coming." Slow-to-warm-up children like to see and talk about the connections between their weekend mini-sessions and their weekday progress. Slow-to-warm-up children are not walking over the bridge if they don't believe the beams are strongly anchored into firm ground.

How can the basic plan be adapted for a child with a difficult temperament?

Like the child with a slow-to-warm-up temperament, the child with a difficult temperament does not welcome change. But unlike the child with a slow-to-warm-up temperament, the child with the difficult temperament is not a receptive partner. She wants it her way and she wants it now.

• Follow your child's lead through the potty preparation process. Give her control over her body and her actions. Creatively add new skills with an invisible hand. Act as if "Potty Weekend," "Naked Noons," or "Potty Play Days" are her idea.

- Present all potty training as a positive. For example, "Is it time to change your diaper?" Use statements rather than requests for your child's participation. For example, "Time to sit on the potty" rather than "Would you like to sit on the potty?"

- Meltdowns during the "Potty Weekend" are expected. Be available to comfort or to pick up the pieces and move forward. Refocus on the goal with clear, simple messages—for example, "Sometimes you don't make it to the potty in time. You will next time."

- Each time you begin "Naked Noons" and "Weekend Mini's," it requires the problematic task of shifting gears for the child with a difficult temperament. A definitive starting ritual is necessary, as is a strong yet compassionate demeanor for you. You may need to allow your child to fall apart or protest without you questioning the course. Simply wait. She will be ready in time (her transition time will get shorter each day).

- If you are the parent of a child with a difficult temperament, plan regular rejuvenating breaks for yourself.

Can I teach my child to poop on the potty before teaching to pee on the potty?

Yes, since the physical sensations of peeing and pooping are different and the ability to control each uses different muscles, your child may learn one before the other. Your child could show an interest in pooping on the potty months before you even start your "Potty Plan."

If your child poops at regular times, incorporate potty time for pooping into your daily routine. This will help him make the potty–poop connection. If your child has both an interest and the physical ability to wait to poop until he gets to the potty, he may prefer to poop on the potty on a regular basis.

The choice is 100 percent up to your child. Once your child learns he can control the sphincter muscles, he has the power to exert that control at will. He can also choose not to poop either in opposition to external demands or in a desire to maintain a sense of security. Always respect your child's choice if he chooses not to poop on the potty.

Should I give my child a diaper to poop in if requested?

Sometimes children completely understand the potty process, and may have even had some initial success peeing in the potty, when they decide they are not ready to poop in the potty. If your child asks you to put on her diaper so she can poop in it, support this need. Reward your child for understanding how her body works and clearly expressing her need. Trust that she knows what she needs.

You can give her the emotional security of her diaper while building her confidence. Give her a verbal affirmation—"I know it feels better to poop in the diaper for now and I know you will tell me when you don't need it anymore."

Continue with your typical bathroom routine. Empty the diaper into the toilet and let her flush the toilet if she wants. Continue to let her wipe herself and wash her own hands.

If your child is older and more verbal, she may be able to explain what she likes about the diaper and what she does not like about the potty. Once you have that information, you can help find a solution to her dilemma.

Given respectful support for her decision, your child will willingly give up the diaper when she no longer needs it.

Should I call potty training a "big boy" or "big girl" behavior?

The drawback to calling potty training a "big boy" or "big girl" behavior is the label. Under ideal circumstances, your child hears the phrase as a positive description of growing-up. But labels can backfire on you. If there's a younger sibling in the house who is a sweet, attention-magnet, being "little" is better than being "big." Your "big" boy might opt for a high stakes negative alternative like deliberating peeing on the Oriental rug.

Focus on "body smart" instead. What does "big" really mean? It means smart, clever, strong, capable, quick, thoughtful, and so on. Talking about "body smart" connects the new skills to your child's body—exactly where you want his attention to be.

What is the best time to start potty training if I am pregnant or getting ready to adopt another baby?

Many helpful people will recommend that you potty train your older child before the new baby arrives. Do not hesitate if your older child is ready. Keep these additional tips in mind:

- Watch out for the pressure of finishing "on time." It's far better to set a solid foundation than to scramble to be completely finished potty training.
- Emphasize potty training time as a positive "together time."
- Make a photo-book for your older child so she can read it when the new baby comes. Your older child

never leaves babyhood behind. It stays within her. Include pictures of her on the potty and a picture of her diaper and her potty chair next to baby's tiny little diaper and changing table.

Do not despair if you do not see readiness traits and you're early in your pregnancy. Pregnancy lasts a long time. If your child is a new two-year-old, the length of your pregnancy is nearly a third of her life span. You have time.

If you're close to the end of your pregnancy and your child is not ready, wait. Wait until the baby is over six weeks old and the household has settled into a comfortable new routine. Enjoy the baby. Give his big sister the opportunity to fall in love, too. Welcoming the baby is far more important than potty training.

Should I start potty training if I am moving into a new home?

If the move is less than a month away, do not start potty training. You have too many other things to do. It is better to use any available free time to hang out with your child—in between packing, that is. Forestall the potty training agenda but continue to immerse your child in a positive potty environment—talking, playing, watching, pretending, and joking. A little attention a few times a day reinforces your potty training momentum. You may start more structured potty training after your child has adjusted to the move, in two to four weeks.

If the move is months away, make your potty training plan with the move in mind.

- Schedule your potty training plan to be finished a few weeks before the move.
- Plan your potty routines so they are easily replicable in your new house.
- Make a My Two Houses book for your child including his old bedroom, yard, neighbors, and your child using the potty in his old bathroom. Add pictures of the new house after you arrive.
- Monitor your stress levels. If you're getting stressed, simplify your plan.

Should I wait to move my child from a crib to a bed during potty training?

Unlike the arrival of a new baby or a move to a new house, the move from a crib to a bed is completely within your control. There's no reason to change sleeping arrangements at the same time you change potty expectations.

If your toddler is climbing out of her crib, you will probably be moving her into the bed before structured potty training begins. If your mellow child is sleeping happily in the crib, daytime potty training can begin while she's still in the crib.

At some point, however, before your child can be potty trained at night, she will need to sleep in a bed so she can take herself to the potty. It may be months or a year between completing daytime potty training and completing nighttime potty training. Choose a time when your child is in a state of developmental equilibrium to make the move to the bed—a time when she has a sense of mastery and is not struggling with any other new skills.

Is it better to wait to begin potty training if we are planning to travel?

Yes, it is better to wait. Potty training is a very child-centered time. The primary focus of potty training days is on bathrooms and your child's body awareness. It's hard to maintain that focus while moving in planes, trains, and automobiles. In addition, the idiosyncrasies of travel bathrooms can be confusing and overwhelming.

However, it isn't realistic to delay all travel until potty training is complete. Simply evaluate the travel arrangements and schedules from your child's point of view. His physical needs and this new skill trump all other adult conveniences.

How can I make potty training easier when traveling?

The secret to successful travel is imagining potty experiences from your child's point of view. Now is the time when all those personal potty routines pay off. Songs and games that can be adapted on the road give your child comfort and confidence. Try to maintain as much consistency as possible with your home routine. Have a plan for your child's predictable potty needs as well as the unpredictable ones.

- Schedule plane flights and layover times accordingly.
- Carry extra clothes, extra pull-ups, and possibly a folding potty seat or a travel potty chair.
- Plan on potty breaks every two hours, and give your child ongoing encouragement and reminders of the new routine.
- Use diapers to prevent accidents when potties will be unavailable for long periods of time. Diapers alone will not create regression.

What can I do when I feel guilty that potty training coincides with seemingly negative events?

Breathe deeply and know that you are preparing your child for the real world. Your child has your loving support. You are personalizing her potty training experience according to her needs. She is learning to be an adaptable and resourceful problem solver.

If you are positive, your child will have a positive potty experience despite any complicating life circumstances. Release yourself from all guilt of imperfection. New babies, new jobs, and new homes are good stresses. Even negative stresses like family illness or divorce are not traumatic to children if you are child-centered and responsive.

Chapter 4

YOUR PERSONAL POTTY PLAN

- How will my life change once I start potty training?
- Am I a positive potty role model?
- What words should I choose for body parts and bodily functions?
- How do I teach my child that some body parts are private when potty training is so public?
- When should I buy a potty chair or a potty seat?
- How do I encourage my child to "make friends" with a potty chair or a potty seat?
- What foods make potty training easier?
- Who should be on my potty team?
- How do I get the potty team on the same page?
- What do I need to gather or buy for my potty plan?
- How should I prepare the potty space?
- What is a "Personal Potty Plan"?
- When should I implement the plan and how long will it take?
- Can I customize my "Personal Potty Plan"?
- What are some positive potty messages to include on the "Personal Potty Plan"?
- What are my child's potty training strengths?
- How should I introduce my child to potty training according to verbal strengths?

■ How should I introduce my child to potty training according to physical strengths?

■ How should I introduce my child to potty training according to imagination strengths?

■ How should I introduce my child to potty training according to social strengths?

■ How should I introduce my child to potty training according to cognitive strengths?

■ When should we switch from diapers/pull-ups to cloth underwear?

■ Is nighttime potty training different than daytime potty training?

■ What is an optimal nighttime potty routine?

■ Will wearing pull-ups at night inhibit daytime potty success?

How will my life change once I start potty training?

When you make the move from casual to structured potty training, your life changes dramatically. Your routines are now child-centered because you are on hourly potty alert. You are thinking for two until the potty process becomes second nature to your child. Simple daily actions now take longer. You are doing "more" during the potty times and you are doing "less" as your child assumes more responsibility for his own body.

• You plan your day around available bathrooms at critical times.

- You give your child the time and opportunity to communicate his needs, to remove his clothes, to wipe after pottying, to wash and dry his hands, and to finish what he started.
- You make time to wait while your child "tries" to potty before transition times—before going outside, before going in the car, before nap, before bath, or before starting any extended activity.
- You plan on the possibility of accidents for at least six months.

Am I a positive potty role model?

Now, more than ever, your child is watching you. She is studying what you do, what you say, and especially what you don't say. She's probably taking notes, too.

- Are you open or secretive about your bathroom behavior?
- Are you following the hygiene routine, too?
- Do you believe your child will be successful in her own time?
- Is potty training a genuine priority or do you fit it in when it's convenient for you?
- Do you talk about your child's potty abilities to other adults in front of your child?

- Do you talk about dirty diapers or soiled clothes as "icky," "yucky," or "nasty"?
- Can you see potty training through your child's eyes to prevent your own boredom and burn-out?

What words should I choose for body parts and bodily functions?

Pee and poop, #1 and #2, bm (bowel movement) and urinate—There are many word choices for bathroom activities, but only a few that you will feel comfortable using on a daily basis. Your choice of vocabulary matters. Your words shape your level of comfort in talking about the potty experience to your child. Choose words that seem natural to you.

Avoid cute and foreign words that will not be recognized by other family members and caregivers. Your child needs to communicate his potty needs to many people, including teachers. You want to choose words that everyone recognizes.

The recommendation for body parts is more specific. Try to use proper names for body parts: penis and vagina. Your child needs to know the proper names even if you use other cute or affectionate terms as well. Remember, your child needs to be able to tell the doctor if and where something hurts.

Preferences are personal and change from generation to generation, so everyone on your potty team may not agree with your choices. Start by knowing, and sticking to, your own preferences.

How do I teach my child that some body parts are private when potty training is so public?

You may hear yourself saying, "That's private," to your child when she doesn't really understand what that means. Privacy is a difficult concept for young children. Socially appropriate boundaries around pottying are ambiguous and probably better left for a time after your child has mastered the potty process. Questions during the potty training process need to be answered immediately, regardless of the potential embarrassment of the adults present. In most cases, a direct public explanation of "We're potty training" should excuse any violations of etiquette.

This is a time, however, to label parts of your child's body (i.e., penis and vagina) as private. That applies to all the body parts covered by a bathing suit. Potty training is the first step in a multiyear process of teaching your child that she owns her body. For better or for worse, she decides what she likes and what she doesn't like. You want your child to believe the power of her own voice, even when she says "You can't make me."

When should I buy a potty chair or a potty seat?

When you see your child starting to imitate your daily actions, somewhere between eighteen and twenty-four months, you can introduce him to the potty chair. The older child who has expressed an interest in using the potty can participate in the selection. Otherwise, select one that you will enjoy seeing in your bathroom for a while to come.

It's personal preference whether you prefer a potty chair or a potty seat to attach to the top of the toilet. The potty chair can be used more independently by your child—it's just the right height, perfect for pretend, and doesn't have the fear factor of a real flusher and real water that make things disappear out of sight. The potty chair also affords your child the ability to plant his feet directly on the floor, which helps him get in position for pooping.

If you use a potty chair, at some point your child will have to make the transition to the big toilet. There's no transition if you choose to begin with a potty seat. In addition, the clean-up is simple. The potty seat is a natural choice for children attracted to the big toilet. Always keep your child's specific interests and personality in mind when you make your final decision.

New products, new designs, and new theme characters regularly appear on the market. Moms and dads everywhere will be happy to share their best and worst purchase decisions—all you need to do is ask.

How do I encourage my child to "make friends" with a potty chair or a potty seat?

Before you begin any structured potty training, your child should be familiar with the furniture. She already knows that she has a high chair or booster seat for eating, and maybe a small table and chair for playing. The next step is learning she has a place to potty just like Mommy and Daddy have a special place to potty. The intellectual and emotional connections are made through casual play.

The first step is "ownership," when she learns, "Look, this is mine!" "Mine" is a powerful word for your toddler. Let her revel in the feeling, especially when something really is hers.

The next step is "appropriate use," when she learns what to do with this new chair. The possibilities are endless. She can sit on her potty chair. She can read on her potty chair. She can play with a doll on her potty chair. However, there are limitations. She may not use her potty chair to climb onto the bathroom counter. She may not throw small toys into the potty chair. She may not use her potty chair instead of a chair at the dinner table.

The "making friends" step comes when she decides, "Yes, I like this." Your child is interested in using the potty chair, spending time there learning about her body and what her body can do. She is not frightened, intimidated, or overwhelmed by the existence of her potty chair.

What foods make potty training easier?

Taro Gomi ends the wonderful children's book, Everyone Poops, with the perfect phrase "All living things eat, so…Everyone poops." Food and pottying go together. Potty training is easier if you are giving your child plenty of fluids and non-binding foods. High-fiber foods keep things "moving." Too much dairy slows things down.

Give your child healthy meals and snacks. Give him plenty of water. Prune juice, peach nectar, and pear nectar ease constipation. Brown rice, wheat and multigrain breads, bran cereals and muffins, fresh and dried fruits, and fresh vegetables all help digestion.

Limit junk foods, high-fat foods, and dairy. Avoid giving your child crackers, cookies, and sweets that fill him up before he eats healthy high-fiber foods. Reduce white flour breads and pastas. Monitor daily amounts of dairy products with milk and cheese. Also, decrease portions of bananas and applesauce if your child is complaining of hard poops or seems to be pushing too hard.

Who should be on my potty team?

Your child's personal potty team includes the primary potty training teacher, the potty training assistants, anyone who will be speaking to your child about her potty adventures, and finally your parent-support people.

Some households may have the luxury of a few candidates for the primary potty training position—stay-at-home parents, work-at-home parents, live-in grandparents, full-time nannies. Choose the person who has the time and the emotional compatibility with your particular child. If, for example, Dad is the parent who has fewer power struggles with the potty training child, then Dad may be the best choice for the job. Then, design your potty plan around Dad's schedule. If the only potty training candidate is the person most likely to get frustrated, try to identify helpful support people to ease parent and child stress.

The assistants on the team will be co-parents, siblings, and anyone else taking your child to the potty. They need to know the potty plan as well as all the tools to guide and encourage your potty training child. You also want to have brief conversations with those friends and family members who will discuss pottying with your child. Let them know the "name" of your potty adventure and your long- and short-term goals.

Pottying can be challenging, so the team ought to include cheerleaders and resources for the parents, too. Add to your list phone-friends who will lend a sympathetic ear during times of regression, experienced parents who will remind you that your child is normal, and pinch hitters to assist when you have a schedule conflict.

How do I get the potty team on the same page?

Good communication brings your team together. First build consensus among everyone living in your home. Remember, you've invested considerable time and energy in formulating a potty plan. You've had time to think about your child's individual personality and to consider a few different potty training options for him. This discussion may be the first time the others have given any thought to the subject of potty training. However, they probably have a few assumptions and expectations from their own experiences. Do not rush ahead in implementing the plan until everyone is on the same page.

Brief everyone, including the extended team. Talk to grandparents and all your potty helpers. Explain your goals and your strategies. Tell them how you'd like them to help. Be specific. If they are receptive, share encouraging phrases and the fun parts of your potty routine. They want to be successful, not frustrated.

Everyone wants what is best for your child—to be successful, to grow in a timely way, and to avoid the physical and mental stress of a negative experience. Reassure everyone that rushing only delays progress. You are the person who knows your child best. Give others your time-proven tips to best support your child.

What do I need to gather or buy for my potty plan?

Potty training is easier if you have everything you need in the place that you need it. If you have what you need, you are also prepared to teach the new routine the first time you do it, which is especially important for those parents and children that thrive on consistency.

- Stock your kitchen with potty friendly drinks and snacks.
- Gather a basket of children's potty books.
- Buy your choice of fun-to-wear pull-ups or training pants.
- Select outfits that include easy on/off clothing (no overalls, no tight clothes, no hard-to-do buttons, and no special care clothes).
- Choose your potty chair or potty seat (are there themes, colors, or styles that appeal to your child?).
- Find a step stool for easy hand washing.
- Add some new theme hand towels or fun soap to the potty bathroom (optional).
- Choose your clean-up product for accidents (extra towels, floor cleaner, disinfectant).
- Pick a place for wet or soiled laundry, preferably a place your child can throw her own clothes as needed.

How should I prepare the potty space?

Choose one bathroom close to where your child plays or sleeps. This may pose a problem if you live in a two-story house. If so, the potty place needs to be close to where you will be spending most of your "Potty Play Day." Or, you have the option of buying multiple potty chairs for multiple bathrooms. Add your step stool and any other fun potty accessories.

Pick a time to show your child "his" new potty place. As you explain your "Potty Weekend" or "Potty Play Days," walk your child to his bathroom and show him where all the action will be happening.

Update child-proofing in the potty training bathroom for your child's new skill levels. If you haven't thought about child-proofing since your child was a baby, you may have overlooked the medicine chest and high shelves that are now easier for him to reach. You may also have to remove toilet locks and put the toilet paper back on the roller.

What is a "Personal Potty Plan"?

You have done your preparation—you know what you're getting involved in, sort of. You've set a foundation for a positive potty experience. Your child is interested in using the potty and she has had some casual success. Now, it's time to look into the future and make a guess of how to bring it all together. This is not an arbitrary role of the dice. You can now make an informed decision based on years of parenting experience.

Will you choose the "Potty Weekend," "Naked Noons," or "Weekend Mini Potty Play Days"?

- Remember temperament styles. Does your child like to go into new situations slow or fast? Does your child need structured routines or can she adapt some to inconsistency? Does your child want to do everything "her way" or does your child prefer a little hand-holding? Does your child get stuck in frustrating situations or barrel forward through frustration? How can you best support your child's chances of success?

- Evaluate your needs. Are you ready for an all-consuming weekend or do you prefer devoting a little time each day? How hands-on do you want to be and for how long? What is realistic given your current work and family schedules? How can you best manage months of potty training activities?

Use the following guide to see which plan best fits your child and your family: For example, the "Potty Weekend" works best for parents who like structure and for children who adapt more quickly to change. "Naked Noons" work best for parents who can maintain consistency for an extended time and for children who like a slow and steady pace. "Weekend Mini Potty Play Days" work well for unstructured parents with full schedules and for children who are extremely adaptable and independent but not for children who need more consistency and structure.

Potty Weekend	Naked Noons	Weekend Minis Potty Play Days
More structured	More structured	Less structured
Depends on previous activities	High consistency	Low consistency
More adaptability required	Low adaptability required	High adaptability required
Faster pace	Gradual pace	Gradual pace
Intense focus	Gentle focus	Gentle focus
More potential for independence	More potential for cooperation	More potential for independence
High frustration potential	Low frustration potential	More frustration potential

When should I implement the plan and how long will it take?

Your potty-age child is most likely in a developmental stage of wanting to know what's coming next. Remember, emotional comfort and intellectual predictability go hand-in-hand. Or, as the adults say, knowledge is power. While you may be ready to begin "tomorrow," your child probably needs a little more advance warning—especially the child with the slow-to-warm-up temperament. The child with a difficult temperament will need "invisible" preparation—that is, without too much talking.

With that in mind, pick a start date at least a week or two in advance. If you're choosing the "Potty Weekend," your ending date is clear but flexible. The part-time potty options require you to look ahead in your schedule. Are other events coming up that disrupt the consistency of your potty plans—holidays, vacations, visitors, new babies, new schools, birthdays? Be sure to plan for and with the expected happening.

Can I customize my "Personal Potty Plan"?

Yes. In fact, you already know who, what, where, when, and how. Formally or informally, construct your plan and make it your reference point for the weeks ahead. Personalize the plan with your child's favorite themes and characters. Plan activities that will interest your child at times that are convenient for you. You don't want to be caught at the end of your "Potty Weekend" without the cupcakes or the right words to encourage your child to the next step.

For those who like the formality of an organizing chart, here is a Sample Personal Potty Plan and a blank form to write your own plan.

SIMPLE POTTY PLAN

We're busy, busy, busy—that's us!
But we still like to play.
Going on the potty is fun. Let's try it today!

WHO	WHAT	WHERE	WHEN	HOW
Mom Dad	Snacks, juices, new cereals	Downstairs bath	Weekend Minis starting June 1 —in two weeks	Slow and steady
Afternoon sitter Date-night sitter	Princess Pull-Ups Princess potty Princess stool Princess towels Princess hamper	Add potty chair one week before on [date]	Practice Saturday mornings and Sunday after naps	Plan pool time Picnic snacks with princess cups and plates
Grandparents Neighbors				
Friend with four-year-old Best friend in Ohio	Spray bottles Cleaner	Remove medicines Take off lock on toilet	Try for one month Ready for party on the fourth of July!	Celebrate Sunday nights with princess cupcakes

OUR PERSONAL POTTY PLAN

Our Positive Potty Message

WHO	WHAT	WHERE	WHEN	HOW

Post your plan in a visible place where you will see it daily. Add some of the positive messages listed in the next question to reassure you when you feel discouraged, to honor the uniqueness of your child and your family, and to keep you focused on moving positively toward success.

What are some positive potty messages to include on the "Personal Potty Plan"?

Sometimes you need a positive affirmation to get you through a challenging potty day. The following messages help when you or your child is frustrated or confused by the potty training process. Keep sight of your long-term goal and revise your short-term goals to be more realistic.

1. Our "Potty Weekend" is the gateway to growing a little bigger. I will give my child my attention and the tools for successful pottying. Soon, we will say good-bye to diapers—"See ya, don't need ya!"

2. Yeah for our "Naked Noons." Take off your diapers and feel how your body works. "I like to practice on the potty—I sit and I try. One day I won't need those bulky diapers to keep me dry!"

3. We're busy, busy, busy—that's us! But we still like to play. Going on the potty is fun. Let's try it today!

4. Hooray for potty days! We eat. We play. We potty. I love my body. Sometimes I like my diaper. Sometimes I like the potty. I always like growing smarter and taller.

What are my child's potty training strengths?

You have a plan. You may have even written down your plan. The next step is to communicate that plan to your child and to the potty team.

Since you want your child's fullest possible participation in the potty process, it's best to pick a communication style that matches your child's strengths. Just as your child is born with a temperament style, he also has personal communication preferences. Although these may be learned or may be genetic, you've probably witnessed them for most of his life.

- If your child was an early talker and is an avid listener to people and stories, one of his strengths may be verbal ability.
- If your child is a physical risk-taker and has boundless energy, one of his strengths may be physical ability.
- If your child enjoys playing with pretend figures and accessories, one of his strengths may be creative imagination.

- If your child lights up around other children and plays well with them under most circumstances, one of his strengths may be social ability.
- If your child enjoys solving puzzles and is drawn to the details in toys and books, one of his strengths may be his thoughtful nature.

How should I introduce my child to potty training according to verbal strengths?

The child with verbal strengths loves explanations. She listens to "the plan," rephrases "the plan" in her own words, repeats key phrases to remind herself what to do next, and gains control over her action by talking. If you are a parent with similar verbal strengths, this is easy and natural for you. If you have other strengths, your child's need for talking can drive you crazy.

Inspire your word-loving child for success in the following ways:

- Give your child simple explanations in advance of the potty process.
- Describe the sequence of the potty process (when/then; 1-2-3).
- Give your child the opportunity to talk, read, and sing about her experiences.

- Create key phrases to capture a positive attitude about accidents and mistakes.

How should I introduce my child to potty training according to physical strengths?

The physically precocious child is a doer who likes to do first and reflect afterwards. You must appeal to his sense of adventure and need for action. If you keep his body busy, you will engage his mind. However, if you ignore his body, he will be bored and distracted. Because potty training requires self-awareness, you must hook the verbal/cognitive message onto predictable actions.

Inspire your physically precocious child for success in the following ways:

- Give your child full responsibility to "do" everything he can.
- Acknowledge every time your child is "on task."
- Be your child's inner voice describing expectations and success.
- Celebrate with "high fives" and an "end-zone dance."

How should I introduce my child to potty training according to imagination strengths?

The child with a large imagination excels at imitation and pretend play. She is observant, engaged, and attuned to the rich details of everyday actions. The imaginative child may embellish play with narrative themes or characters. Some children may assume new identities or include imaginary friends.

Inspire your imagination-driven child for success in the following ways:

- Incorporate themes and characters on your potty equipment.
- Make pottying fun with games and rituals.
- Create opportunities to rehearse potty skills in pretend play.
- Use favorite theme characters to support and encourage mastery.

How should I introduce my child to potty training according to social strengths?

The strengths of a little social butterfly have been obvious from the first time he left your arms for another's. He makes eye contact easily and encourages social connections just like any great politician.

He initiates and welcomes social interaction. He'll happily be the last to leave the party. He learns best with others rather than alone.

Inspire your socially dynamic child for success in the following ways:

> - Teach by example and recruit positive role models.
> - Keep the cheerleaders near and vocal.
> - Invite your child to join the "club" of his potty-going peers.
> - Be an active potty partner by giving your child your time and attention.

How should I introduce my child to potty training according to cognitive strengths?

Your mini-intellectual loves sitting still and figuring out how things work. She may be one of those children that seems wise beyond her years. She enjoys working on logical puzzles and games (for example, sorting, sequencing, matching, and counting). She may also love books and self-designed science projects (for example, what happens if I take this apart or if I mix this with that?).

Inspire your curious cognitive child for success in the following ways:

- Use engaging questions to reinforce the sequence of the potty process (for example, first we "feel it," then we "go to it" or bathroom 1, 2, 3—potty, wash, hooray!).
- Make pottying a game where everything is in its rightful place and everything is in order.
- Help your child to be flexible when things don't go the "right way"—explain there's more than one right way.
- Give your child the opportunity to figure out her own solutions to problems.

When should we switch from diapers/pull-ups to cloth underwear?

Underwear is a big milestone in the potty game. Try not to be too anxious to make the switch. Your child will get his long-awaited underpants after he's demonstrated he can stay dry with ease. If you don't feel fairly confident that the majority of potty training is behind you, don't do it. You want Las Vegas house odds that your child is mastering the potty routine. He has the skill and he has the attitude to say, "See ya, don't need ya!"

After the practice of the "Potty Weekend" and "Potty Play Days," the move to underpants is a definite good-bye to diapers. Not maybe, not cross your fingers, and not a bribe. Sometimes your child cannot resist the lure of underwear and he'll make promises he can't keep—"Please Mommy, please Mommy, pleeeeease." In this instance, you know better than your child if you're setting him up to fail. If the skills are not there, underwear won't make a difference.

There are times when the switch to underwear brings the final click to the potty puzzle and it's worth the gamble. If your child is overly cautious about change or risks, you may have to lead the way. Just be sure you're ready to live with the consequences. You will need to be a positive, supportive, hands-on potty partner if you make the switch and your child is not ready, willing, and able to go it alone.

Is nighttime potty training different than daytime potty training?

Many children are potty trained during the day long before being potty trained at night. Readiness for daytime potty training is not a sign that your child is ready for nighttime potty training. The sign to start nighttime potty training is seeing your child wake-up with dry diapers on a regular basis.

Your child needs two physiological abilities to master nighttime pottying: She needs to hold her pee for a longer period of time and to wake-up if she needs to pee in the middle of the night. Awareness, control, and interest all work hand-in-hand. If your child is a deep sleeper, she won't have the awareness. If she doesn't realize the need soon enough, she may not have the control. If her bedroom is far from the bathroom, she may not have the interest.

Fortunately, your child can sleep in her favorite character pull-ups without any physical discomfort or troublesome anxiety. The American Academy of Pediatrics says nighttime potty mastery may not occur until four or five years of age. Speak to your pediatrician if you have any concerns.

What is an optimal nighttime potty routine?

Your child's nighttime success has much to do with your pre-bedtime routine. It's up to you to make good decisions for your child. Your potty training child is too young to comprehend the consequence of drinking too much late in the day. And if he understands the connection, he is too young to delay the gratification of enjoying that last glass of water.

Stop drinks a few hours before bedtime. Make a potty stop the last thing you do before the last good-night kisses. If you have an extended tuck-in routine with multiple stories, you may allow your child that one extra trip out of bed. Watch out, however, for hourly requests to use the potty after lights out—chances are these are clever ways to capture your attention and not really about pottying at all. Finally, be clear about what your child should do if he needs to potty. Choose a routine appropriate for his age and abilities. Do you want him to call for you? Do you want him to walk to the bathroom? Which bathroom? Are there any other "rules," like "And go right back to your bed"?

If you notice your child is usually dry at night, there might be a simple explanation for the occasional wet night. It might have been the night your child fell fast asleep driving home from his grandparents and never made the last potty stop. If everything seems the same as on his dry nights, just relax and wait. Check with your pediatrician if your child starts having nighttime accidents after six months of nighttime mastery.

Will wearing pull-ups at night inhibit daytime potty success?

Attitude is everything. Wearing pull-ups at night frees your child from the pressure of mastering something that is temporarily beyond her ability. Waking up in a wet bed is very unpleasant and has no ultimate teaching value.

Explain to your child that she can wear her underpants at night when she wakes up dry in the morning for a week or two. Do not add the pressure of counting the calendar days with her—this is not a situation that needs external motivation. Night wetting is about physiological maturity.

Focus on how good it feels to sleep in something that keeps her and her bed dry. Take full advantage of the fun pull-up products on the market. If you are okay with nighttime pull-ups, your child will be, too.

Chapter 5

ACCIDENTS, SURPRISES, AND MISTAKES

- How do I teach a boy not to shake pee on the bathroom walls?
- What if my child plays with her poop?
- How do we handle nighttime accidents?
- How long should my child wear pull-ups at night?
- Should I change my child quickly after an accident or delay for a few minutes?
- How many accidents are too many?
- What if my child asks for a diaper now and then?
- Will accidents upset my child's self-esteem?

Do most children have potty accidents?

Potty training is a long-term process that is often three steps forward and two steps back. In many cases, the two steps back aren't regressions. They are simply your child learning to generalize what she knows in a variety of new contexts. Your child may have easily mastered her "Potty Weekend," only to discover that different people, different places, different sounds, different routines, and different moods all affect potty success.

Potty training does not end abruptly after the "Potty Weekend" or "Naked Noons." It is a gradual transfer of responsibility from you to your child. When your child was a baby, you took full responsibility for her pottying. When she was a young toddler, you immersed her in new potty experiences as she watched and imitated you. When she expressed an interest, you created a potty time just for her. After a few consistent successes under her belt, you still "thought for two" but gave your child the opportunity to act on her own. Now, you will teach her to stretch those skills, to adapt to the unpredictable, to conquer age-appropriate fears, and to learn from mistakes.

You should expect accidents for a few months after your "Potty Weekend," "Naked Noons," or "Potty Play Days." Accidents may even occur sporadically through the preschool years. Young children forget and young children make less-than-perfect choices. An understanding, supportive response will prevent a minor accident from becoming a major issue.

When are potty accidents most likely?

Imagine yourself in the body and the mind of your potty-going child. Your child's inner world looks and feels very different from the one you know. Sometimes your child gets all mixed up. Sometimes his head knows what's right while his body is doing the opposite.

Accidents are likely when your child is busy. Your "Potty Weekend" was finely focused on potty-going behavior. Your child had ongoing reminders. The entire day revolved around making pottying fun and easy. Now, real life adds hundreds of distractions—an interesting video, a bug he's never seen before, or the last bite of a cookie. Young children have difficulty stopping whatever it is they are doing, even if that thing will be waiting there when they return. It isn't rational, but it's the way children think.

Accidents are likely when something is different than expected—Dad uses different words when he gives a potty reminder, the potty chair is in the wrong place, or your child is startled by the dog. Your child shifts his intellectual and emotional focus to comprehend the changes and whoops...he forgot what he seemed to know so well.

Accidents also happen because your child has an immature sense of time—how long it will take to finish something, get to the potty, and take off his clothes. Potty-age children frequently underestimate time.

The reasons for accidents are as numerous as hours in the day. It's a wonder children ever manage with all the possibilities. Your child may be sick or in a bad mood, or you may be sick or in a bad mood. Using the potty might seem like such a bother today.

Whatever the reason, accidents happen. Expect them.

What should I do when my child has a potty accident?

What do you want people to say to you when you make a mistake? "Why did you do that—you know better!" "That's it, lady—no birthday party for you!" "I told you that would happen!" Blame and humiliation are counterproductive in potty training. Negative emotions discourage future success and prevent your child from finding a better alternative.

Your child still needs you as a supportive partner who is keeping her focused on her goal. You want your child to be a potty pro—resourceful when faced with the unexpected, motivated despite obstacles, and adaptable in imperfect conditions.

1. Check your emotions before you speak or act. You may be tired, discouraged, frustrated, angry, confused, desperate, worried, and just plain overwhelmed. It's okay—you're normal. Hold that thought and call your potty-support friend later. You're entitled to complain and scream a little, just not at your child. Your child cannot and will not learn while you're in an emotional state.

2. State the situation in neutral terms for your child. Simply describe what happened. For example, if you're out shopping and see your child standing in a puddle with a nervous look on her face, you can say

"I didn't know you needed to use a potty." This helps your child focus on what happened instead of any negative emotions. Keep in mind—your child literally may not know "what just happened." She hasn't processed it yet. She's wet, physically uncomfortable, possibly embarrassed, and is wishing she could close her eyes and make it all go away.

3. Find a solution. Problem solving aloud helps your child become a problem solver, too. "Let's find a bathroom where we can change your clothes. Not to worry, I always bring extra clothes for you just in case we need them." Or, "We don't have extra clothes with us today. That's okay; we'll drive home to get some." Sometimes, even the all-wise, all-knowing parent has no idea what to do. Here's your chance to be a truly great role model. When in doubt, stall. Just say, "Hmmm, I wonder what we should do now?" Let the world stop around you until you think of something.

4. Be positive. Leave your child with the hope that she can be successful. Let her know you are confident that she will succeed, too. Laughter is also powerful medicine for mistakes—just be sure you are laughing with, not at, your child.

Is it possible that my child is having accidents because he knows it annoys me?

Most of the time, your child's accidents are genuine mistakes. It is possible, however, that your child's behavior has become a game, particularly if you have allowed your emotions to rule your reactions. When children learn that they can push parents' buttons, they are almost compelled to do so. It gives them power, albeit inappropriate power. They can pull you into an ever-escalating emotional drama. They get attention—they win, in child-logic anyway.

One sure way out of the game is to neutralize your emotional response. Take a time-out. Count to ten. Count to fifty. Here's one script for a hypothetical situation.

Describe: "I see you pooped on the carpet again and (I see) you are laughing about it."

Problem solve: "I'm not laughing, and I want to clean up the floor before we do anything else."

Be positive: "This isn't fun for me. You can tell me in other ways if you don't want to use the potty."

The next step is to continue the problem solving about the accident. The game is often initiated during one of those oppositional stages in development when your child is strongly asserting his independence. If so, explain to your child that it is not okay to choose the floor instead of the potty. If the action was attention-getting, the behavior will stop when you are not emotionally engaged by the action.

As much as you might like to, you cannot force your child to use the potty. Although you may be angry at your child's willfulness, the best long-term strategy is always to pull back from the struggle. By doing this, you will shorten the oppositional standoff and prevent escalating misbehavior.

Should I scold my child for having an accident?

The potty training process has enormous potential for negative emotional interaction. Potty training is emotional for the child because it requires feeling secure and confident. It requires self-awareness and self-control, both of which are extraordinarily complex for potty-age children. When the experience is difficult, a child may want to withdraw or give up, which may be done quietly or vehemently.

The potty training process is equally difficult for some parents. It revolves around a very personal balance of parent–child control and is a very public measure of child development.

Scolding heaps more emotional complexity into the mix. It's so much better to focus on skill building.

Harsh criticism distracts your child from her goal of success and detracts from your effectiveness. When you scold your child, you are communicating strong disapproval as a way of motivating a different behavior. You are adding the unnecessary threat of fear and rejection to a teaching situation.

You don't have to resort to such extreme measures. You cannot win this game if your child chooses to exert retaliatory control. And you do not want to win if your child is left feeling bruised and battered.

What is a natural consequence?

There are times when you allow your child to experience the natural consequences of his actions. Peeing in his underpants feels uncomfortably wet. Pooping in his pants makes them smell, so he'll need to change out of his favorite pants. Accidents on the floor need to be cleaned up. He still needs to wear diapers or pull-ups at night until he can stay dry for a week.

Your child may not like these consequences. However, they present problem-solving opportunities for your child. They are age-appropriate dilemmas—difficult life lessons that things don't always go the way you want them to go. These consequences are necessary for growth.

One of the hardest jobs in parenting is letting your

child learn from experience. Give your child the tools to overcome frustration and disappointment rather than trying to avoid, or protect him from, negative consequences.

What is the difference between punishment and a natural consequence?

There is no inherent emotional drama connected to a natural consequence, which is why natural consequences are important teachable moments. Threats and punishment throw you and your child into an emotional tug-of-war that interferes with potty training.

Avoid the following emotionally laden phrases:

- "You don't like wearing wet pants, do you?" said tauntingly.
- "I'm not buying you any more underpants if you can't stay dry."
- "You can't go to the park with your friends if you don't go on the potty right now."
- "That's it. If you have one more accident, I'm throwing away all your underpants."

Threats and punishment are acts of parent desperation. Understandable, yes, but also counterproductive. Stay calm. Describe the situation. Find solutions. Have faith in your child.

What do I do if someone else belittles my child for a potty accident?

Here you are, maturely controlling your own emotional reactions, and along comes someone else who believes your child just needs a good old-fashioned push in the right direction. Your response depends on how involved the guilty person is in your family life. If the person is a casual acquaintance, explain that you disagree with her motivational style. If she righteously persists, spend a few months apart until you finish the potty training stage and surround yourself with your supportive potty team.

If the person is a close friend or family member, you may have to invest a little more time and energy in the problem. Ask the person to stop while explaining the success you are having using positive potty messages. Help that person find better words to use with your child. Remember, it takes years to learn respectful communication with young children.

Should I ask my child to help clean up after an accident?

Yes, let your child be part of the solution. It will teach him a sense of responsibility, just like if he wipes up spilt milk. Clean up together. Cleanup is not coercive or a form of punishment. Make cleanup a game, but be sure to let the grown-ups handle any actual poop cleanup.

- Keep it light. "Whoops, I think we have a cleanup here!"
- Ask for help. "I need a handy helper here!"
- Make helping easy. Keep supplies (paper towels, a nontoxic cleaning solution, a change of clothes) in a child-accessible place (on a low shelf or in a basket in the bathroom).
- Lead the way. Start the cleanup if your child resists, acting as if he's a full participant: "We'll have this problem fixed in no time at all."
- Avoid long lectures. Let the natural consequence do the teaching for you. Only speak about "woulda, coulda, shoulda" if your child initiates it.
- Practice good hand washing afterward.

Should my child empty the potty chair if she makes more of a mess?

Children love to help, and they rarely see their efforts as causing more work for adults. Taking responsibility for the potty chair is a continuation of your child taking responsibility for her body. Follow your child's interest here. If she wants to do more, she will be learning valuable self-sufficiency skills that will make your life easier next year when she's more capable at the details. Try not to worry about perfection—accept small approximations at careful assistance.

Discourage recklessness. Potty training and bathrooms are supposed to be fun, but they are not a free-for-all. You may need to slow down overly zealous helpers. Remind them that splashing the pee makes more to clean up. If you sense your child is playing more than helping, thank her for her effort and give her something else to do.

Children evolve into competent helpers through routines and experience. Coercion only leads to conflict. As mentioned earlier, there is no room for conflict in successful potty training. If your child is not a willing helper, wait until after potty training to add this extra skill.

What can I do to help my child remember to use the potty?

After your "Potty Weekend" or your "Naked Noons," gradually turn over the responsibility to remember to potty to your child. Of course, depending on your child, this transfer might be fast or slow. The best strategies to give your child ownership over his potty training experience are ones that keep your involvement as invisible as possible.

- *Use routines*. Create new habits for your child by incorporating potty stops into natural daily transition times. Routines are one reason why preschools are so successful at potty training. Everyone takes regular preventative potty breaks. What are the optimal times? When your child first wakes up, before he gets dressed, after breakfast, before all car trips, when you arrive in new places, and before beginning involved activities are all optimal potty times. Keep in mind that you can't force your child to potty. Never insist that he has to actually potty—only state matter-of-factly that these are times to "sit and try," just in case.

- *Use signals*. Children need gentle—as in non-nagging—reminders. Verbal reminders are fine, but feel free to be creative, too. Draw a "P" with a question mark on your child's back when you think it's been a while since his last potty break. Give a "T" for a potty time-out.

- *Use games*. Incorporate a bathroom game into the potty plan. Add a whiteboard or chalkboard to your child's potty place where he can give himself a checkmark for sitting on the potty. Or, you can add a bell to your child's potty place and he can ring it when he's been successful. Of course, when you hear the bell ringing, you will cheer, too!

What if my child is always last minute–too late?

What if you've given your child all the appropriate reminders and she's still dancing the potty two-step in the family room when she should be on her way to the bathroom? Let it be her accident. That might sound completely avoidable and unnecessary to you as an adult, but you already know how to use the potty. If you could make your child's potty choices, the potty training process would be infinitely easier. However, some children need to find out for themselves.

Maybe your child is playing a game with her body to see how long she can wait. Maybe she wishes she could play for five more minutes and then go. The situation will change as soon as your child doesn't like the outcome. Stay calm. Be patient. This problem won't last forever.

What if my child jumps off the potty before he is finished?

Some children are always in a hurry. They run fast, eat fast, and potty fast. If your child is interested in using the potty but is too impatient to sit still, you may want to incorporate some delay tactics. Sing a song together, read a story, teach him to whistle—anything that will help your child to slow down.

In the meantime, treat the accident like any other accident. Let your child be aware of the near-miss and clean it up without too much fanfare. His initial impulsiveness should not lead to deliberate carelessness. With more experience, he will learn to be more careful.

If your child starts to pee on the potty, then stops halfway through and finishes peeing in his pants, he may be less than 100 percent sold on the potty process. Watch for excessive external expectations. Let him wear pull-ups until he's more willing to use the potty. He may need more time to become a trusting friend of the potty.

What if my child goes on the potty when naked but has accidents when wearing underwear?

Your child has not been able to connect the skills she learned in one situation into the larger context. She needs more time without the stress of frequent accidents. One reason could be that she "reads" her body better when naked. If so, only have her wear underpants in controlled settings at home when you are as prepared for the accidents as when she is naked. You might return to "Naked Noons" to recreate the optimal practice setting. Explain that she needs to wear her pull-ups when you are out or when it's not a "Potty Play Time" because you want her to have fun doing all the other things she loves to do.

Another reason for the difference is that using the potty may not be a high priority when your child is dressed and actively engaged. The accidents are a signal to you to back up a few steps. Unless you want to be a hands-on potty partner actively anticipating your child's needs, you are better off waiting for increased self-motivation. When she truly cares, she'll get there.

Is it normal to have accidents after months of potty success?

Many children will have accidents after months of successful pottying. There are many reasons why your child is having accidents. He forgot. He got scared. He made a bad choice. After months of success, he is probably very aware of his mistakes. Potty training is emotional, and your child may have lost his previous sense of control.

Hold your doubts in check, particularly in front of your child. Continue to observe the situation for changes in your child's environment. If the situation doesn't improve, contact your pediatrician or speak to your child's teacher. But for now, wait and watch. Acknowledge the situation with acceptance and address the immediate problem—a change of clothes and a hand to hold. Reconfirm your faith in his ability.

What do I do if my child is seeking out unusual places to poop?

Children can find very creative places to poop—behind the sofa, in a closet, under a tall plant. Look at the bright side: At least you will know where it is. Your main objective is to help your child feel comfortable using the potty. If you chastise her potty place, she won't be persuaded to trust your choice.

She will not understand if she's being criticized or humiliated.

Re-establish the connection between the poop and the potty, just as you would if your child was asking to poop in a diaper on a regular basis. Let your child see you taking the poop to the toilet and flushing it down. Do this without scolding, theatrics, or emotional hoopla.

If you see your child going to her private place to poop, gently try to bring her to the potty. If that causes tremendous stress, however, allow her to continue. Try to make her chosen location as sanitary as possible. Invite your child to help with the cleanup.

How do I teach a boy not to shake pee on the bathroom walls?

Many potty behaviors draw adult shrieks and/or laughter. Most of you will have potty stories for each of your children that will, and should, become family classics. Boys are notoriously messy when it comes to peeing on or at a potty. They spray, shake, and dribble. At times, you may grow impatient with the constant mess. Other times, you may be laughing at your little man growing up so quickly.

Always evaluate your reaction before trying to teach your child considerate bathroom habits. If you screamed, "Watch out for the walls!" the first time your child shook before he finished, you inadvertently drew your child's attention to his awesome range. And now, instead of being more careful, he may need to verify his latent skills for the Potty Olympics. The same is true for laughter—it will be much harder to refrain after your child has found his audience.

Try to remain low key. Quietly clean up the accidents. After beginning potty training, your bathroom is no longer an adult sanctuary. It is better to repaint and regrout than to lose a child-friendly atmosphere.

What if my child plays with her poop?

Why would a child play with poop? Because it's there. Plus, she has yet to learn all of the negative associations that you have. It's gross, but so are boogers and spitballs. Gross isn't much of a deterrent to children.

If your child discovers the playful qualities of poop, be prepared to be extra watchful in the days and weeks ahead. Poop may have a self-reinforcing attraction to your child—it's soft and squishy and smears well. An emotional response on your part ("Ooooh gross," "Stop, that's disgusting," or "Yuuuuuuuck") also reinforces the behavior. It could create a greater interest to play with poop.

Stay calm in front of your child. Scream, laugh, or cry with your potty-support friends. Describe the problem: "Poop belongs in the potty. It has germs. So we don't touch it with our hands. And that's why we wash our hands every time we use the potty." Fix the problem: "Let's clean this up." No scolding is necessary if you clearly present what is okay and what is not okay to do with poop. Because poop may hold a unique attraction to your child, allow for the possibility that this is not a one-time experience. You may have to repeat your message a few more times.

End with a positive. If your child loves to get messy or loves ooey, gooey textures, incorporate more of those things into her play. Try squishing play dough, finger painting with paint or pudding, mixing a bowl of flour with a pitcher of water, digging in the garden, or making mud pies.

How do we handle nighttime accidents?

Nighttime accidents are more difficult to handle than daytime accidents because your child may not have the physical control to be successful. Plus, everyone is obviously tired. That said, try to handle nighttime accidents the same as daytime accidents, with a calm problem-solving perspective.

If your child is sleeping in underpants and having infrequent accidents, you can minimize the inconvenience with a plastic mattress cover. Let your child know that it's no big deal to wash the bedding, especially if it's once in a while. He already feels bad enough waking up to an unexpected mess.

Attend to his emotional needs as well as his physical needs. Reassure him that the accidents are isolated instances; they will not happen every night. Listen to his worries and help find solutions together.

- Gently talk about the situation with an older child. Does he feel like he has to pee during the night? Is he willing to get out of bed to potty at night? Make sure your child is clear about what he should do. Add night lights, floor "runway" lights, or a nearby nighttime potty chair.

- Review the nighttime potty plan. Add an extra potty time before you go to bed and first thing in the morning. Would your child prefer calling for you in the middle of the night? (Is this okay with you if it happens once a month?)

- Reconsider bedtime routines. Have you been more lenient lately about those late-night potty reminders? Does he say he'll stop in the

potty after reading his books and then fall
asleep instead? Is he drinking more?

- Evaluate daytime routines and changes. Are
you or your child busier lately? Is he adjust-
ing to some new challenges? Maybe you
need to plan ten minutes of game time to
just hang out together after dinner.

Reassure your child that you will help him stay dry
at night and this is a problem you will conquer
together. If you are still worried, contact your pediatrician to eliminate any medical causes.

How long should my child wear pull-ups at night?

The physiological components of nighttime potty-
going may not be there when you or your child are
ready. Your child may be motivated to get out of the
pull-ups but still not be able to hold her pee for the
duration of the night. She may also not wake up if
she feels the need to pee. She may be frustrated by
unrealistic expectations. You may have to be the "bad
guy" by explaining that it's not time for nighttime
underpants until she wakes up dry for one week.

Delaying the switch to underpants is preferred
over ongoing weekly failures. Time is on your side.
Many parents are surprised to hear that a significant

number of four- and five-year-olds still have night-time accidents. There's no shame to wearing nighttime pull-ups. Keep nighttime expectations separate from daytime expectations and make the switch to full-time underpants after more long-term nighttime success.

Should I change my child quickly after an accident or delay for a few minutes?

If your child comes to you after a potty accident seeking your help, you should respond in a helpful way. Communication is a key ingredient to potty training. The physical and emotional desire to be clean and dry is a powerful potty motivator. At the same time, your child is looking for your help and approval, which also further your potty goals.

If you notice your child has had a potty accident and you are wondering what he might do next, you may take a few minutes to observe your child's interest and problem-solving abilities. If your child truly doesn't care, you may want to rethink the timing on your potty training and wait a little longer. If the diapers or pull-ups are interfering with your child's physical awareness, you may choose more naked time. You may also find your industrious little potty-goer may attempt to fix the situation all by himself.

You should not use the delay tactic as a means to blame or shame your child. You will undermine your child's faith in you as a reliable potty partner. Blame and shame are unproductive emotional messages in potty training. Your goal is to increase your child's ability to fix mistakes. Disapproving emotions simply cloud his ability to problem solve in a very age-appropriate situation.

How many accidents are too many?

While you did your best to make a one-way switch to underpants, there may come a time when you decide to change course. Possibly the readiness behaviors just aren't there, your child has reached a new oppositional stage, or family circumstances have changed the positive dynamic. The original plan has become too frustrating for you or for your child.

Daily accidents for several weeks are too many. Your child is showing you she doesn't want to do this. Step back. Explain to your child without any blame or shame that you decided it will be better to wait for another time. Wait a week, or a month. Keep a positive potty atmosphere until your child is ready to make a fresh start.

What if my child asks for a diaper now and then?

The answer to this question is directly related to your potty training personality. Can you be flexible without losing faith? Can you introduce a little inconsistency without confusing your child? Can you say "no" while still acknowledging his underlying need?

Try to understand what lies behind his request. Is there a new sibling in the house? Is your child having doubts about growing up? Is this a request for attention or for reassurance? Attention without reassurance will lead to more requests for attention and escalate the situation. Attention with reassurance will meet your child's needs and allow him to continue to move forward.

Choose the response that feels right to you:

- Say, "Okay, just this one special time." Have a follow-up conversation with your child. "Why" questions are difficult for three-year-olds to answer, so try to explore the situation in other ways. Instead ask, "How does it feel to wear the diaper again?" or "Do you want a break from thinking about the potty?"
- Use humor and play to redirect the situation without laughing at your child. For example, "I don't have any more diapers.

Let's make pretend diapers out of paper towels and put them on your teddy bears."

• Address the need in other ways. Sometimes it's not about the diapers but the ambiguity of growing up. Validate the need with simple words like "I loved it when you were a baby and I took care of you all the time. Let's plan some special time for just you and me." Then add a morning snuggle time together, time each day to look at baby pictures, take an evening walk, or go on a Saturday afternoon ice cream outing.

Will accidents upset my child's self-esteem?

Your child develops healthy self-esteem by learning she is capable. She knows she has skills and personal strengths. She also knows she is resourceful in times of trouble and people want to help her succeed. Mistakes are invaluable to building healthy self-esteem. A child who learns not to fear mistakes has nothing to fear.

Children who meet with quick success are not always well-prepared for situations that require adaptability and problem solving. Instead, they can be easily discouraged by adversity and delayed gratification. You might wish you could protect your child from frustration and disappointment, but then she will not know she is fully capable. Instead, she might believe that she couldn't handle the situation.

Potty training is a complex achievement in your child's development. In the end, you want your child to say loud and clear, "I did it!"

Chapter 6

TRICKS, TREATS, AND GIMMICKS

- How can I create a positive potty bathroom?
- Do potty training pull-ups make potty training easier?
- Is it okay if my child likes to read books on his potty chair?
- What books and videos should I choose for my child's potty library?
- What are some favorite children's books and videos about the potty?
- How does pretend play help facilitate a positive potty message?
- Do potty training dolls make potty training easier?
- What is a personal My Potty Book?
- How do I make a personal My Potty Book?
- When is praise a positive potty strategy?
- Can rewards be a positive potty strategy?
- When are rewards not a positive potty strategy?
- Are stickers and charts helpful potty tools?
- Should I use food as a positive potty strategy?
- Can I use music as a positive potty strategy?
- What are some favorite children's potty songs and music?
- How do I encourage my child to sit long enough on the potty?

- What tricks can help improve a boy's potty aim?
- What are some positive potty bathroom games?
- What are some fun "underwear" books, games, and songs?
- What are some positive potty clean-up games?
- What are some positive potty games for nighttime trips to the potty?
- Which commercial products will make potty training easier?
- What are some favorite potty training resources?

How can I create a positive potty bathroom?

Some children will happily potty anywhere at any time. But for other children, a bathroom is a formidable place with big, hard fixtures and big, cold expectations. Your first trick in potty preparedness is making sure the bathroom is a happy place for your child.

You don't need a professionally decorated child-themed bathroom to entice your child. You definitely do not need expensive fixtures and accessories that have you hovering over your child's use. What does your child look at when he sits on the potty? Would he like a mirror to see himself? Would he like to see a piece of his artwork framed or an enlarged picture of himself on the potty or of him washing his hands? Would he like a book basket nearby? Look at your potty room from your child's point of view and create a place of ease and comfort for your child.

- Write your child's name with a colorful permanent marker or add stickers to his potty chair or his step stool.
- Add theme towels or personalized name towels. Decorate on your own with fabric paints, check out your local flea market, or buy him something special online.
- Use child-friendly hooks for your child's towel instead of the usual towel bar.
- Add some fun foam soap in an attractive child-pump dispenser.
- Create a pull-up/dry clothes station where your child can change during the transitional weeks. Designate a drawer or add a cubby for clean pull-ups.
- Double-check that the temperature on the hot water is turned down.
- Use an easy-to-wash enamel-base paint on the walls.

Listen and stay aware—even though your child is becoming more independent in his potty time, continue to supervise when he's in the bathroom for safety and for positive potty habits.

Do potty training pull-ups make potty training easier?

Potty training pull-ups may increase your child's self-awareness by giving her visual or sensory cues when she potties in her diaper. Some children will be attracted to the newness of the experience as well as to the child-friendly design. Potty training pull-ups are also fun interest-generating tools for potty training.

Keep in mind the biggest challenge to potty training is your child's awareness before she potties, then her ability and motivation to choose the potty instead of the pull-up. While potty training pull-ups assist you in the potty process, you still need a potty plan to guide your child through to mastery. Potty training pull-ups cannot create physical control where none exists.

Potty training will always be the push and pull between convenience and mess. Accidents may be messy but they are the mistakes that teach. Although you may choose convenience, there are no shortcuts.

Is it okay if my child likes to read books on his potty chair?

Young children love to read on the potty, especially if they have potty reading role models. Your child will imitate you. Reading may also help your child sit on the potty longer. Keep a basket of books, catalogs, and old mail next to your child's potty, but also let your child know that potty reading is a means to an end and not an end in itself.

Allow your child to sit on the potty with his books as long as he likes during the "making friends with the potty" stage. This is the time when your child is building familiarity with the fit and feel of his potty. Once he has that confidence and understands the purpose of sitting on the potty, give him gentle reminders of why he's there. It's okay to wait for a poop or a pee, but you don't want him sitting there reading indefinitely. Distinguish between playing on the potty and purposeful potty behavior.

What books and videos should I choose for my child's potty library?

The majority of books in your child's potty library basket will be her preferred classics and her rotating library selection. However, your child does need a few fabulous books specifically about pottying. One favorite that is full of potty content but has no potty training agenda is *Everyone Poops* by Taro Gomi. This book is exceptional as a biology book for little people. It is the science of a child's body as expressed by the phrase "All living things eat, so...Everyone poops." It is the perfect first potty book because there are no emotional expectations for a child to resist. And what child doesn't laugh when you read the final page, "Everyone poops"?

Choose books and videos that your child likes. Just like adults, different children will connect with different books and videos. Children will choose a book or video because of their own personal criteria. The illustrations or the photographs might tell the whole story, or the singsongy language might grab them. Other times, it's the image of a little-girl queen or a child who looks just like them. Some children want the silliest potty book in the world while another child wants an emotionally triumphant potty adventure. You don't have to buy them all, however. Take your time to find your child's favorite. Buy your favorite, too.

Having a few meaningful books and stories at your child's fingertips whenever she wants them is one more way of giving your child power and ownership over her potty experiences. Read ahead for some favorite potty titles.

What are some favorite children's books and videos about the potty?

Favorite Children's Potty Books:

- *A Potty for Me!* by Karen Katz
- *Does a Pig Flush?* by Fred Ehrlich
- *Everyone Poops* by Taro Gomi
- *Go, Girl! Go Potty!* by Harriet Ziefert Inc.
- *Going to the Potty* by Fred Rogers
- *I Have to Go!* by Robert Munsch
- *Lift the Lid, Use the Potty* by Annie Ingle and Lisa McCue
- *No More Diapers for Ducky* by Bernette Ford and Sam Williams
- *No Potty! Yes, Potty!* by Harriet Ziefert Inc.
- *Once Upon a Potty* by Alona Frankel
- *The Prince and the Potty* by Wendy Cheyette Lewison
- *The Princess and the Potty* by Wendy Cheyette Lewison
- *The Potty Book for Boys* by Alyssa Satin Capucilli
- *The Potty Book for Girls* by Alyssa Satin Capucilli
- *Time to Pee* by Mo Willems
- *Uh Oh! Gotta Go! Potty Tales from Toddlers* by Bob McGrath

- *What Do You Do with a Potty?* by Marianne Borgardt
- *Where's the Poop?* by Julie Markes and Susan Kathleen Hartung
- *You Can Go to the Potty* by William Sears, MD, Martha Sears, RN, and Christie Watts Kelly
- *Your New Potty* by Joanna Cole

Favorite Children's Potty Videos

- *Bear in the Big Blue House* by Martin Hugh Mitchell
- *I Can Go Potty* by Mazzarella Productions
- *It's Potty Time* by Learning Through Entertainment, Inc.
- *Let's Go Potty* by Dr. Betti Hertzberg
- *Once Upon a Potty for Her* by Alona Frankel
- *Once Upon a Potty for Him* by Alona Frankel

How does pretend play help facilitate a positive potty message?

Children integrate what they learn into personal experience through play. That's why repetition is abundant during the potty learning years—children ask to read the same books, just like they often wear the same clothes and rely on a particular bedtime routine. Giving your child the opportunity to playfully reenact potty behavior builds confidence and competence. He mentally rehearses and problem-solves different potty scenarios with dolls, teddy bears, books, songs, and videos.

- Let your child pretend by holding a doll or teddy bear on the potty. Listen to how your child speaks to the doll to get a glimpse of what he's thinking.

- Buy real baby-size diapers. Set up a pretend diaper changing station where your child can re-experience diapers with a doll or bear. Though your child is leaving his diapers behind, he can re-live his emotional connection to diapers through play.

- Use hand-puppets, finger-puppets, or spoon-puppets to have a conversation about potty training. At first, you can speak for the mommy and the child puppets, telling a story about a little boy who was learning to use the potty. In time, you and your child can switch roles and incorporate any new potty themes that arise in your home.

- Extend your child's favorite potty stories and songs into everyday play situations. Retell the stories from books and videos while you are driving in the car or walking to the store. Comprehension increases with every retelling.

Be sure to casually supervise the "play potty" situations. You don't want your child really peeing on the doll's play potty and you don't want the teddy bear sitting in real pee. Treat either of these as you did an accident in the last chapter. Stay calm. Explain what's okay and what's not okay. Fix the problem and end with a positive. If your child is confused between real and pretend, feel free to remove the play props until a later time when your child understands the difference.

Do potty training dolls make potty training easier?

Children who are learning to make the connection between what comes out of their body and what goes into the potty may enjoy seeing a potty doll that actually pees in the potty. Potty training dolls teach children the immediate cause-and-effect connection between drinking and peeing. Some dolls pee immediately after drinking while others do not pee until their stomach is pressed.

This is one piece of the potty puzzle. However, successful potty training occurs when all the developmental pieces are in place. If your child loves playing with a potty doll, you are creating a meaningful positive potty environment. The potty doll may be the perfect addition to your potty plan.

Consider your individual child. What does your child understand about her own body and other potty role models? Does she already understand the connection between pee and potties? Dolls can play a significant role in the learning process. You decide whether you need a doll to make a literal connection to the potty or whether your child's imagination can do the trick.

What is a personal *My Potty Book*?

Your child's personal My Potty Book is his potty story. The more specific it is to his needs and his journey, the more perfect it is. Your child loves looking at himself. To a potty-age child building his self-image, pictures become one way to define who he is in the world.

Photo-books increase your child's self-awareness. He can reflect on the images and think, "Aha, that's what I look like." He might discover that the potty isn't so big, or he might feel pride sitting on the potty reading his book or seeing himself flushing the toilet, remembering that it was a little scary the first time.

Photo-books increase your child's potty comprehension. Books are tangible. It's easier to remember the potty sequence when you see it in a book in front of you. A photo-book takes abstract potty choices and makes them concrete for your child. Your child can read his potty photo-book any time and anywhere—when he's happy, proud, frustrated, sad, or confused. He can read it alone or with someone else. Books have power. A potty photo-book gives your child power.

How do I make a personal *My Potty Book*?

1. Take six to ten potty pictures. If you have more pictures that you want to include, divide them into two different potty-theme books. You want each book to be short and sweet. Here are some suggestions for pictures and captions. However, feel free to customize your books your way:

> a. A picture of your child wearing a diaper ("Once upon a time I wore a diaper.")
>
> b. A picture of your child playing ("I can feel it when I need to use the potty.")
>
> c. A picture of your child going into the bathroom—waving, smiling, and generally acting it up ("Got to go!" or "Got to go. Now!")
>
> d. A picture of your child sitting on the potty

("I feel good.")

    e. A picture of your child washing her hands ("Happy potty to me…")

    f. A picture of you kissing, hugging, or high-five-ing your child ("Yeah, I did it!")

    g. Additional pictures might be of different bathrooms, the potty without your child on it, a teddy bear on the potty, friends and family cheering for your child, or an artistic still-life of underpants on display on a clothesline or in an interesting arrangement on the bed.

2. Paste or print your pictures on heavy card stock paper.

3. Write or print your captions. Fewer words are better for these young readers.

4. Decorate the book with stickers or designs, if desired.

5. Laminate it at your local office store.

6. The My Potty Book is to be well read and well loved. Your child's book will become worn and battered. Make two if you want a keepsake to put away. You should also make additional copies to keep at a grandparent's or baby-sitter's home.

When is praise a positive potty strategy?

Praise is sincere positive feedback you give your child when he does something well, makes good choices, or strives to learn a new skill. Praise is a personal gift of recognition from you to your child. The best thing about praise is you always have it when you want it.

As your child's potty training partner, your meaningful praise guides your child toward greater success. Praise tells your child that he really is on the right course. It gives him the encouragement to keep trying. Your child doesn't always know that those small potty successes really will lead to being diaper-free. Right now, diaper-free is beyond his personal reality, but not yours.

Praise also discriminates between successes and mistakes. Praise for the sake of praise is meaningless. It doesn't teach skills and doesn't build self-esteem. Rah-Rah praise just leaves your child wondering, "Hey, if I was doing it right, why am I still stuck in the same place?" He will feel much better having you as the problem-solving partner than a short-sighted cheerleader.

Praise your child every chance you get. Be sincere. Tell him what makes you happy. Tell him what makes you proud. Honor him and his success with your words and your actions.

Can rewards be a positive potty strategy?

The most effective rewards will emphasize your child's accomplishments instead of the stuff. The best rewards give your child the messages "Hooray for ME" and "I did it!" They reinforce the positive potty partnership and the thrill of success.

Time together is always the best reward. Quick token rewards are the substitutes in a fast-paced, move-on-to-the-next-thing-on-the-to-do-list world. Give your child the real gift of stopping to give attention to something well done. Incorporate daily and weekly rituals to commemorate your child's journey into this strange new territory:

- Plan mini-celebrations with cupcakes and a potty candle-lighting ceremony.
- Create a photo wall of happy potty pictures.
- Call friends and relatives with positive potty reports.
- Plan a grand finale ritual when you finally say good-bye to diapers—dance around a trash can as you throw away the last diaper, have an underwear party where everyone wears silly underwear over their clothes, flies underwear-wearing helium balloons, or has a parade waving underwear on sticks.

Daily potty games can also be rewarding to children. If you incorporate games that immediately capture your child's interest, you don't need additional external rewards. Potty training can be a positive experience by itself. It isn't something your child must do in order to earn a better prize.

When are rewards not a positive potty strategy?

Rewards are tangible tokens commemorating your child's accomplishments. Most children love getting stuff. The problem is that potty-age children do not always remember the symbolism of the gesture. They get hooked on the stuff and forget that this toy or those candies were about making good potty choices. Your child may see the reward as an end in itself.

Then, your oh-so-smart child realizes the game and decides to work it to her advantage. Instead of increasing long-term potty success, your child becomes skilled at negotiating for bigger and better rewards. Can you see her now, hands on hips with her toe tapping "Oh yeah, you want me to sit on that potty—where's my ____?" Unfortunately, what began as a positive potty training partnership has become an escalating power play with your child. You are held hostage by your child constantly looking for the right pay-off.

Are stickers and charts helpful potty tools?

Stickers and charts may be positive activities that record your child's growing skill at pottying. You can make a weekly poster from poster board with long column spaces for daily stickers counting your child's potty times (see the following chart). Let your child put a sticker on his chart when he uses the potty. Your child's active participation in a sticker activity is his personal announcement that "I did it!"

This activity can also be done by drawing "potty stars" using whiteboard markers and a whiteboard or chalk and a chalkboard. Whichever you may choose, keep the chart in the bathroom for immediate follow-through.

Monday	Tuesday	Wednesday	Thursday	Friday	Saturday	Sunday

A potty chart is better as a child-directed activity than as a parent reward system because it gives your child personal ownership over his success. An external expectation to "earn" stickers or "potty stars" can create the same power struggles as token rewards and praise.

Should I use food as a positive potty strategy?

Food can be a positive ingredient in rituals and celebrations. Focus on the event and the joy of being together. Plan a trip out for ice cream or let your child eat homemade sundaes naked on "Potty Play Days." Remember, it's one thing to teach children the spirit of generosity by giving them things they like. It's another to withhold what they like unless they do something you want. Potty training cannot be conditional—that will only teach your child to perform on demand. Your goal is to teach your child to understand and trust her body.

Using food as a reward can have negative consequences. Children can begin to make emotional connections to food that can follow them into their adult lives. As with other token rewards, children can easily confuse the piece of candy as the goal instead of the "Hooray for me—look what I can do!" Your child is not being trained to do "tricks." If she could learn to walk without the lure of treats, she can also feel proud and capable in her body without token treats. Potty training is prime time to concentrate on your child's positive attitude about her emotions and her body.

Can I use music as a positive potty strategy?

Music helps children internalize the positive potty message in the same hands-on way as books and pretend play. In addition, children grasp the information at a deeper level when language is combined with music. Singing routine potty songs also reinforces positive potty training.

Use songs:

- For transition times
- To help an active child sit still
- To focus your child on a specific potty skill like hand washing or walking to the bathroom at night
- To give emotional encouragement

Read ahead for a list of children's potty songs and music. You only need a few favorites to do the trick. Pick a melody and a message that feels just right for singing on a daily basis. Learn one or two that make you smile and enjoy the silliness of being a potty training partner!

What are some favorite children's potty songs and music?

- *Miss Joanie's Potty Party* by Joanie Whittaker

- *The Once Upon a Potty—Potty Songs* CD by Ari Frankel
- *Potty Animal: Funny Songs about Potty Training* by Auntie Poo & The Porta-Potties
- *Potty Song: Customized Potty Training Song* at www.pottysong.com
- *Potty Song 1*, *Potty Song 2*, and *Potty Song 3* (free potty songs) on www.pottytraining concepts.com
- *Tinkle, Tinkle, Little Tot: Songs and Rhymes for Toilet Training* (book) by Bruce Lansky, Robert Pottle, and Friends

How do I encourage my child to sit long enough on the potty?

Fun and games are better encouragements for your child to sit on the potty than bribes or coercion. As usual, continue to create a positive potty experience and avoid any power struggles. Look for strategies that teach an active child how to slow down and an impatient child how to wait. For some children, these are important skills that need to be practiced, and are not their natural tendency. The following suggestions are things to do while your child is learning to tune-in and control her potty muscles. Use them to buy your child some time to be successful but not as a distraction from her ultimate purpose.

> • Play "I spy" describing things you see in the bathroom. End with "Do I spy something in the potty? Yes, I do!"
>
> • Play "I hear" describing things you hear in the bathroom, in the house, or outside the bathroom window. End with "Do I hear something in the potty? Yes, I do!"
>
> • Sing one of your favorite potty songs from the preceding question. Or try this one adapted from "Here We Go 'Round the Mulberry Bush":
>
>> This is the way we sit on the potty,
>> Sit on the potty, sit on the potty,
>> This is the way we sit on the potty
>> Early in the morning.
>>
>> (every afternoon/early in the ev'ning/before we go to bed)
>
> • Customize your own "Fast Boy" story:

Once upon a time there was a little boy who everyone called "Fast Boy." He was fast, fast, fast—always running and jumping, never sitting still. When he wanted to learn to use the potty, he would fly in and out of the bathroom so fast. He flew right over his potty. His mommy had to think of some way to help him sit long enough to use the potty. Fast Boy's mommy talked to the queen of the bees, who had many fast little bees. Queen bee gave Fast Boy's mommy a special sticky potion that would catch Fast Boy on his potty. And from now on, Fast Boy's mommy always covers Fast Boy's potty with the mixture from the bees. Do you feel it? I think there's some on your potty right now.

What tricks can help improve a boy's potty aim?

Accurate aim is a skill that requires focus and coordination, and it comes with experience. Practice may not make perfect, but at least you can make it more fun. Sometimes you can improve your child's aim just by sitting him backwards on the regular bathroom toilet. Otherwise, try some of these classic adaptations:

- Play "sink the cheerio."
- Add blue food coloring to the water and watch it turn green when the pee hits it.
- Buy commercial animal-shaped tissue paper "toilet targets" and "training urinals."

What are some positive potty bathroom games?

All children like games. Children who generally do not like change like potty games because they create a familiar ritual around the newness of the potty experience. Pick one of these simple potty games to add to your child's potty routine. Don't try every one of the following suggestions—just sample a few of the ones that sound genuinely fun to you or your child.

- Laminate homemade "red light" and "green light" cards that your child can put into a decorated tissue box in the bathroom. "Green light" if she went potty, "red light" if she did not. You can also use smaller "red light/green light" cards with Velcro on a bathroom poster board.

- Make a handprint of your child's hand on a bathroom tile or poster with the words "High Five." After your child sits on the potty, she can stop to give herself a "high five."

- Draw a happy face on the bathroom mirror every time pee or poop makes it into the potty. Use Crayola® washable window markers or any brand that can be washed off when potty training is over.

- Sing a potty song. Here's one to the tune of "Frere Jacques":

  Are you peeing? Are you peeing?
      Little one? Little one?

Yes, I am. Yes, I am.

Now I'm done. Now I'm done.

- Collect toilet paper rolls. Use them for horns, tunnels for small cars, or a background to paint on. Line them up and count them.

What are some fun "underwear" books, games, and songs?

Underwear is fun and funny. Take advantage of your potty training time to cultivate your "underwear" theme repertoire. Every parent needs a high HQ (i.e., "humor quotient") to make parenting easier. When it comes to underwear, there's no better time than now. Celebrate wearing underwear with enthusiasm. Let your playfulness reinforce your potty goal—saying good-bye to diapers is fun!

Who knows, you may be creating a family-time ritual that will last for years.

- Add the books *Underwear!* by Mary Elise Monsell and Lynn Munsinger, or *What Color Is Your Underwear?* by Sam Lloyd, to your home library. Congratulate your child as he becomes a member of the underwear-wearing club.

- Buy extra large underwear to wear over clothes or even on your head. Wear for "underwear parties" or for "underwear dancing." Or go for the "world's largest underwear" that the whole family can all wear at the same time.

- Collect your favorite dance songs for daily "underwear dancing." An "underwear" favorite is Joe Scruggs singing "Big Underwear," available on the *Ants* CD.

What are some positive potty clean-up games?

Believe it or not, children like to clean—if clean-up is a game. The most effective strategy is to be ready before accidents happen. Eliminate the "uh-oh" factor. Have the clean-up supplies in a convenient location. Teach your child how to be helpful. Gently supervise until your child knows the boundaries between helpful and not-so-helpful. Generally speaking: If your child is "trying," it's helpful (you may need to stand near with an extra towel). Continue to encourage good hand washing and let your child "spray clean" after you pick up the poop accidents.

> - Spray bottles always make clean-up more fun. Buy a small spray bottle that fits your child's small hands. Practice outside or on

mirrors with plain water. Be sure to fill with a non-toxic, child-friendly cleaner.

- Sing a clean-up song. It can be one you already know or an invented potty version. Here's one to the tune of "Old McDonald." Substitute your child's name for David:

  Little David cleaned the mess.

  E-I-E-I-O.

  With a wipe wipe here and a wipe wipe there.

  E-I-E-I-O.

  Little David cleaned the mess.

  E-I-E-I-O.

  Choose words to fit any situation:

  Little David sprayed the spray.

  Little David wiped the floor.

  Little David pitched the trash.

- Buy an inexpensive plastic wastebasket with a flip-flap cover and draw a "hungry" face on the flap. Name your potty "trash-eating" animal.

What are some positive potty games for nighttime trips to the potty?

Beds are very comfortable places when you're sleepy. Your child may wake up with the sensation of needing to potty but it might still take enormous effort to actually get out of bed, especially when he's small and it's dark. If your child is having difficulty getting to the bathroom, practice some of these bathroom games during the day to build his nighttime confidence.

- Make a masking tape line from his bed to the potty.
- Trace his footprints on construction paper. Cut, laminate, and tape a path to follow on the floor from his bed to the potty.
- Put a fun flashlight by his bed to shine the way.
- Add a song to the walk. "Heigh Ho! Heigh Ho! It's off to potty I go!"
- Count the steps from his bed to the potty during the day. See if there are more or less steps at night.
- Talk about all the animals that come out at night—smart owls, strong tigers, quiet snakes, noisy crickets, sneaky sharks. Let your child pretend he's one of those animals when he wakes to go potty. (Remind him to go right back to bed though.) Give him a nocturnal pet like a gerbil or horseshoe crabs.
- Add a Johnny-Light to the toilet and your toilet will light green (for "go") when the toilet lid is up.

Which commercial products will make potty training easier?

Luckily, you live at a time when the market tries to make potty training as easy as possible. Take advantage of these creative solutions but remember that successful potty training is about your child's personal skills, personal motivation, and her positive potty experiences. Potty training is not about the right stuff—the stuff is just a tool.

Don't buy everything. Survey parents near and far. Ask them what they'd never want to live without and ask them about the biggest waste of money. As expected, one person's essential is another's mistake.

Start the potty training with your potty chair or potty seat, your choice of pull-up, some children's potty books, and your fun bathroom accessories. Follow your child's lead as you add to the accoutrements. If your child is older and wears pants with belts, by all means buy a Velcro potty training belt. If your child loves Dora the Explorer, buy a folding travel potty seat with Dora the Explorer on it.

What are some favorite potty training resources?

Retail stores large and small now carry a wide range of helpful potty products. Check out your neighborhood

Babies-R-Us, Baby Love, K-Mart, Target, Toys–R-Us, and Wal-Mart. Online searches bring numerous potty training resources right to your fingertips. The following list of popular websites offers a wide range of potty training supplies. It is not an endorsement for a particular site or any specific potty training supplies, nor is it comprehensive of all vendors.

Through browsing the sites, you will discover potty supplies that are fun, helpful, and/or extravagant. You will find potty seats and chairs in every size and shape, in every color and theme (from animal characters to TV characters), as well as features to suit any personal lifestyle, from flip-up home attachments to cushioned folding travel seats. You will also find potty training dolls, games and calendars, watches, targets, mattress covers, and step stools. Enjoy yourself as you discover that you are not the only parent hoping to find the right potty training combination for your child.

- www.babycenter.com
- www.babylove.com
- www.babiesrus.com
- www.companystore.com
- www.pottytrainingconcepts.com
- www.pottytrainingsolutions.com
- www.onestepahead.com

If you're looking for the "Johnny-Light" for the toilet that lights up green when the toilet lid opens, check out www.johnnylight.com or www.pottytrain ingsolutions.com.

For a selection of night lights and "light-the-way" night light systems, visit www.onestepahead.com.

If you're looking to spruce up your bathroom for potty training, check out bathroom accessories at www.target.com and the wall mural at www.wards kids.com. You'll find personalized towels for your child at www.warmbiscuit.com and www.appledoodles.net.

If you must have the "world's largest underwear," check out a local clown supply store or visit www.silly farm.com. And don't forget the Joe Scruggs *Ants* CD with the song "Big Underwear," available at www.amazon.com or at www.hellojoe.com.

Happy shopping—Happy potty training!

Chapter 7

FEARS, STRESS AND SETBACKS

- Are potty fears normal?
- Should I eliminate the source of my child's potty fears?
- How should I respond to potty fears?
- What do I do if my child is hesitant about the move from a potty chair to a toilet?
- What can I do when my child is fearful about flushing the toilet?
- What do I do when a toilet has an automatic flusher?
- What if my child will only use one bathroom?
- What if my child is afraid of using public toilets?
- What can I do if my child is hesitant after painful poop experiences?
- What if my child is afraid of pooping in the toilet?
- What can I do if my child is "withholding" poop?
- How long should my child sit on the potty if nothing is happening?
- What if pottying becomes a power struggle?
- What if my child uses the potty at home but not at school?
- What if my child uses the potty at school but not at home?
- Is it ever okay to lie to my child about potty training?

- ■ Is it okay to push my child if I know he's ready?
- ■ How can I encourage my child to talk about a potty problem?
- ■ What if my child is hesitant about asking other adults for potty help?
- ■ How can I help if my child has an embarrassing potty experience in public or at school?
- ■ How do we resume potty training after a setback (vacation, new sibling, new school, divorce)?
- ■ What are the co-parenting strategies when parents absolutely disagree about the potty training plan?
- ■ How do I respond to criticism about my potty training methods?
- ■ When should I consult with a pediatrician about potty concerns?

Are potty fears normal?

Fears are a normal part of childhood. Fears might be a small isolated moment when your child is face-to-face with something unfamiliar. A simple explanation, a helpful suggestion, or a hand to hold might be all your child needs to move forward. Sometimes all your child needs is a familiar context—"Hey, this toilet looks different than ours. Look at all the ways it's the same as the one in our bathroom." Rational support can help in situations where the fears are specific and clear.

Other times, fears are deep and developmental. The potty training years coincide with a time of sweeping emotional growth. The deepest fear may not be the toilet at all—it may be the more developmental struggle with separation. Separation struggles recur all through childhood as your child grows slowly and steadily into a person—sleeping, crawling, walking, pottying, going to school, and making friends.

Young children often cannot express new complex emotions verbally and rationally. Your child cannot calmly say, "I'm afraid if I fall in that big toilet, I'll slip into the drain and never see you again." Or, as one three-year-old told her mother after weeks of distress, "I want to wear my diaper to bed because I don't want to get old and die."

Before you can calm your child's fears, you must grow comfortable with your own. Children have to face some fears in order to grow emotionally. It isn't easy to see your child struggle, but it is necessary.

Should I eliminate the source of my child's potty fears?

If there's a simple solution to a fear-inspiring situation, by all means use it. But you cannot and should not eliminate all sources of fear. The fear may have little to do with the particular situation and everything to do with your child's sense of power and control. It is better to teach your child that he can handle the situation—he is strong, smart, and capable. Of course, telling him so doesn't make it so. You must give him the tools to face these age-appropriate problems.

When rational explanation fails, you can create routines that pump up your child's power reserves. Routines and rituals transform the unknown into something safe and predictable. Your child is no longer a small person in an out-of-control situation. Your child is the master of his world.

Potty training is an emotional accomplishment as much as it is a physical accomplishment. Addressing fears as they arise will teach your child potty flexibility and all important adaptability. It's big world out there, and it's full of potties.

How should I respond to potty fears?

Responding to your child's potty fears is as easy as ABC.

> • Acknowledge—never dismiss a fear as trivial or nonsense. Your child's fear may not be rational to you as an adult, but it always adheres to the standards of child-logic. You may not know where it originates. It may contradict good sense. But it is "real" to your child. Respect what your child feels with a compassionate adult perspective.

- Balance your response between comfort and power. Your child has an adult partner by her side, someone who can sincerely reassure her that she is safe and capable. It's a fine balance: too much "safe" and you slip into an overprotective mode, robbing your child of her skill-building; too much "capable," and you rob your child of the emotional growth that parallels the behavioral growth.
- Conquer together or alone. Every fear is an opportunity. Solutions will be personal, but there must be some sort of resolution. When possible, let your child decide what to do. Present your child with a few options—sometimes she just needs help knowing what to do next. Then she can conquer the fear "alone." Sometimes, she's willing to act but needs your hand or the physical reassurance that she is not alone. Other times, you will have to act "alone" but with her watching as you act as a brave and resourceful role model.

What do I do if my child is hesitant about the move from a potty chair to a toilet?

The move from a potty chair to a full-size toilet is a big step. Some children have had their eye on the toilet from the first day of potty training. They know what they want to do and they will find their way. But other children may have thought the potty chair was theirs forever.

First, acknowledge the problem. Describe the situation so your child can put the problem in words— "You're right. The toilet is bigger than your little potty chair." Talk about everyday things that are big and small. Make this a math puzzle. Add a little humor. "Do little bottoms fit on big toilets? Oh no…do big bottoms fit on little potties?" Get dramatic. "What do we do if a little bottom falls into a big toilet? We might scream! We might cry! We might say heeeeeelp!" If your child is verbal, all this talking might help him take control of his experience.

For some children, talking about the toilet won't be enough. You will need step two—balance. They need a more emotional response. Build confidence slowly. Add an emotional dimension to your problem solving. Use a doll or teddy bear to rehearse the experience. Explore fears through pretend play. If teddy falls in and gets a wet bottom, show your child how you will hold him and comfort him.

It may take time to conquer the fear. Your child may need to think about it, play with it, or experiment with using the big toilet. You may buy different potty seats that feel just right or that entice your child to make a change. Time spent facing a fear is never wasted.

What can I do when my child is fearful about flushing the toilet?

Plenty of children have fears about flushing the toilet. No wonder—it contains noisy, swirling water that whisks everything away, never to be seen again. It's fast, efficient, and inexplicable. And that's without mentioning that what it takes away is something the child "made." Flushing is scary.

Acknowledge your child's feelings by trying to verbalize the source of her fear. Choose your words and watch your child's body language. You will see her body relax a little when you get it right. For example: "Get ready…here comes the LOUD flushing sound," or "Round and round the water goes, until the bowl is empty at last," or "You don't like that flusher, do you?"

Try to find the balanced response where you recognize your child's distress and find the least disruptive solution. Will your child watch as you flush the toilet? Is it easier if she doesn't watch the contents empty? Make it a game to close the toilet lid, say "Abracadabra," and then check to see if everything is gone. Or simply explain that you see that flushing scares her so you will flush it later—no problem. You might even talk about how scary it is in neutral settings, such as while on a walk or riding in the car. Tell stories and pretend to flush the toilet over and over.

Conquer the problem either alone or together— your child can stand back while you flush, she can wave bye-bye or count 1-2-3 flush, or you might visit the water treatment plant to understand the mystery of where the poop goes. Sometimes a new potty routine makes flushing less frightening. Sometimes your child learns to understand the complex and invisible system of flushing. Or, you may have to be patient and supportive as your child builds confidence slowly.

What do I do when a toilet has an automatic flusher?

Flushing fears become worse when your child discovers some toilets accidentally flush before he has time to get off. Public auto-flush toilets create a new set of fear-inspired drama. Stay with the ABC response, but add new games to build confidence and control.

Do everything you can to minimize the surprise. Make it your public potty routine to check stalls for auto-flush features. Again, potty-age children love high drama. Assume a John Wayne posture and a tough-guy voice, "Okay, we're coming in and we're not afraid of you flushers." Pretend to shine a flush-checking flashlight, "I know you're there and I know when you're going to flush." Keep your child engaged in the power play. Then, help him to prepare for the auto-flush—again by talking to the flusher, "Okay flusher, no flushing until I'm ready. I'm counting 1, 2, 3." Your child learns firsthand to be brave in the face of his fear.

What if my child will only use one bathroom?

Even if you do your best to create a potty routine that is easy and flexible, your child may still insist on using one bathroom. This works fine during the initial training time, but it makes daily errands, school, and vacations impossible. Build your child's confidence step-by-step, taking home skills into an ever-widening assortment of places.

- Use "portable" routines to create familiarity in other bathrooms—potty songs, potty stories, or a teddy bear who always tries the potty first.

- Prepare your child. Guess what different bathrooms will be like and role-play your child's potty experience in different contexts.
- Have a Plan B. If your child still refuses, don't make it a test of wills. Bring diapers, pull-ups, or a portable potty. Think ahead, though—you have to be willing to live with your Plan B indefinitely.
- Be a good role model. Show your child that you are happy and comfortable using a variety of bathrooms, even if you don't really have to use the bathroom.
- Conquer one bathroom at a time. Tell your child to pick one new bathroom each week and keep adding new bathrooms until it's no longer an issue.

What if my child is afraid of using public toilets?

Public toilets require enormous adaptability from a child. Your child must generalize everything she's learned and apply it in situations where toilets, stalls, and bathrooms all have a different look and a different feel. The learning process requires your child to go from a very specific skill of pottying at home, to a general one of pottying anywhere at any time. For some children, this is learned step by step, bathroom by bathroom.

Try to keep your potty routine as consistent as possible. Show your child she's doing the exact same potty steps, just in a different place. Remind her of all her successes. You might even light-heartedly tell her she's used this bathroom before and describe how she did it. Be patient. Although one day your child will make the intellectual and cognitive leap to seeing all bathrooms are more the same than different, right now her focus is stuck on the differences.

Also watch for any negative messages you might be giving about public bathrooms being dirty. Your child cannot feel comfortable if you're grossed out and worried about nasty germs.

What can I do if my child is hesitant after painful poop experiences?

Some children only have to experience a negative situation one time before they learn to avoid it. That helps if you're teaching that the stove is hot, but not when potty training. Try to explain to your child that there is a reason for the hard poop. Monitor your child's diet so you can guarantee easy pooping. It may take lots of encouragement and multiple successes for your child to overcome the negative association between poop and pain. In the future, try to avoid the problem through diet and exercise.

An older child may understand simple explanations of how the body works. Food is the fuel that makes the body go—it builds bones, muscles, and brains. You can explain that pee and poop is what's left after your body takes all the good stuff it needs. But sometimes the poop gets hard and it hurts to push it out. Tell your child that you have good foods that will make the poop soft, and then it won't hurt. Or explain that you have good medicine from the doctor that will help.

Unfortunately, if your child had a negative experience, it may take a number of easy successes before your child lets go of that fear. Use the ABC response: Acknowledge and accept that this hurts. You must be very gentle while encouraging your child to attempt something that caused him pain in the past. In this case, you balance emotions and information when you earn your child's trust that you have food or medicine to help him do something he doesn't want to do. Finally, your child must conquer this one. Watch your emotions because you don't want your child to feel pressure from you. You can encourage and support, but your child is the one who must release this fear.

What if my child is afraid of pooping in the toilet?

Sometimes a child will have all the other potty training skills but still ask for a diaper or a pull-up to poop in. The diaper or pull-up allows your child to relax. This emotional security is essential when pooping. Your child can be "emotionally ready" to pee in a potty or even to stay dry through the night, but still need more time to feel "emotionally ready" to poop in a toilet. If so, be sure to empty the poop from the diaper into the toilet and let your child participate in the rest of the potty routine—wiping, flushing, and hand washing. Reassure your child with a positive message that "One day she'll be ready to poop in the toilet like Mommy and Daddy" and to let you know when she wants to try.

If your child is not asking for a diaper or pull-up, use the ABC response to help your child feel safe "letting go" on the toilet. Acknowledge the situation. Start with a general description like, "I see you don't like pooping on the toilet." Wait to hear if your child can say what you can do to help her feel better. Balance your support by listening for the deeper emotional fears and offering gentle solutions. If your child is feeling like a part of her body is falling off or being taken away to a mysterious place, she needs time to comprehend the process. Here's where flushing the poop from a diaper or the potty chair helps her gradually accept the new potty reality. A balanced response allows you to respect your child's emotions while still taking baby-steps forward. Conquer the fear by telling your child that you can figure this out together. Sit with her, make a game of listening for the poop to fall into the water, and use your other "potty games"—like telling stories.

Of course, the reason for the problem might be a physical difficulty with pooping while sitting on the toilet. Be sure your child can plant her feet firmly on the ground—otherwise, she may be having difficulty pushing the poop out.

What can I do if my child is "withholding" poop?

Like the child in the last question, some children get "stuck"—they know they don't want to poop in the pull-up, but they are still frightened by the alternatives. Unfortunately, getting emotionally "stuck" can lead to getting physically "stuck." Potty training is not fun or easy when your child is constipated. If you've done all the proactive strategies of a healthy high-fiber diet with lots of fluids, have physically active playtimes, and you notice your child is not pooping regularly, check with your pediatrician. Do not give your child over-the-counter laxatives or medicines without your pediatrician's approval.

In a positive potty environment with no medical conditions, your child's body will work as it should. Young children should not depend on laxatives and stool softeners. Use the ABC response to help your child get "unstuck."

Pooping is 100 percent your child's domain. You cannot force him. He might even decide your "gentle encouragement" is excessive. Therefore, acknowledge that he controls when he poops. He must own his potty experience. Withholding situations can be very emotional for the parent and child. Acknowledge your own feelings of frustration and helplessness with your pediatrician or with a non-suppository-recommending potty training buddy.

Balance your response by relinquishing your control over your child's pooping as you help him find appropriate ways to exert control in his world. Show your child all the ways he has constructive control by giving him more choices: what he wears, what books he reads, what characters are on the bathroom towels. Make your response as invisible as possible. Keep potty experiences positive while you try to create more relaxing conditions: add poop-friendly foods, simplify your child's daily schedule, make potty trips easy and unthreatening, and conclude each day with a quiet snuggle time when you re-establish an unconditional connection with your child.

Conquer the problem. Express your faith in your child's ability to do what's healthy for his body. Explain that you don't want him to hold in the poop because it can make him sick and it hurts his body. With positive potty conditions and your relaxed support, your child can enjoy his body again.

How long should my child sit on the potty if nothing is happening?

Younger children who are "making friends" with the potty may sit on the potty for quite a while, looking at books or checking out how their new chair feels. Once your child is in the habit of using the potty, there's no reason for her to sit there if nothing is happening. This could be a signal to ask if your child feels constipated or has any funny feelings from a urinary tract infection. Don't rush your child, but don't let her sit there all day, either.

A child should never be forced to sit on the potty against her will. Do not tell a child to stay on the potty until she potties. You want to avoid creating a negative potty experience and avoid potty power struggles.

What if pottying becomes a power struggle?

Sometimes normal developmental testing behavior spills over into the potty training process. Your potty-age child may not have the self-restraint to avoid escalating conflicts, so it's up to you to be the voice of calm. Power struggles pit you against your child at a time when your child needs respectful guidance on her side.

- Stay calm, at least while in the same room as your child. Try something like, "Instead of fighting, I'll be back in two minutes. Then we can figure this out."

- Let the "rules" speak instead of your authority. For example, "Everyone has to wear a pull-up or underpants in the store. Which one will it be?"

- Substitute gentle reminders for harsh directives. Avoid statements like, "Put those pants on right NOW!" Instead offer the choice, "Two more minutes to get your pants on and then I'll be in to help you."

- Do not give choices when you don't mean it. Instead of "Do you want to go potty before getting in the car?" try in a singsongy voice, "Time for pre-car potty pit stop!"

- Give lots of empowering choices when you do mean it—when both choices lead your child to the desired behavior. For example, hop or skip to the bathroom, Superman underwear or SpongeBob underwear.
- Shut down inappropriate "power surges" quickly. For example, if your child is ready to throw the potty chair, take it calmly and place it out of reach.
- Be ready to say what you want your child to do, not what you don't want. For example, "Let's relax and take a minute to regroup." Or, "We need to walk to our car. It's hard to think with so many people watching us."
- Expect more tantrums as your child releases excessive frustration. Have a tantrum plan to contain hurtful behavior—designate a place where your child can fall apart without hurting himself or being destructive.

Power struggles are never fun. Just remember, testing behavior is a necessary part of healthy development—that is, when the parents don't fall apart, too.

What if my child uses the potty at home but not at school?

Your potty team includes your child's teachers and caregivers. While there may be differences between pottying at home and pottying at school, communication is the key to managing those differences. You want to know as much as possible about the potty routine at school.

- What time do the children potty?
- Do the children go potty as a group or individually?
- Is the teacher near the children or at the door?
- How does the teacher talk to the children about successes and mistakes?
- How do the other children talk about successes and mistakes?
- How is your child doing in non-potty-related school activities?

Any differences from home can create resistance to pottying at school. Stay positive about the school and about the teachers as you help your child adapt her home skills to this new world-away-from-home.

- Give your child time if she just started a new school, has a new teacher, or is in a new class. She will master the potty part of her day after she masters the other changes.

- Share your home strategies with your child's teachers to create a familiar experience for your child. For example, the teacher might enjoy singing your child's potty song or reading your child's My Potty Book.

- Build trust in the teacher. Your child might not understand that the teacher is ready and willing to help. For example, "Ms. So-and-So can help you with your pants. Just tell her when you need her…and be sure she's listening when you talk." Try role-playing if your child is hesitant.

- Ask the teacher if your child can potty last if she is overwhelmed by a group of children in the bathroom. Another option is to have your child taken solo.

- "Write" your child encouraging notes that can either be put in her lunchbox or delivered by the teacher at potty time. Make it reader-friendly by copying some home/school potty pictures or just a big "I love you" heart.

- Give potty reports back and forth from school to home. Keep it light—"just checking." Let your child see that you and the teacher are working together in a positive way.

Some schools will adapt to your child's potty needs while others will ask your child to adapt to the school routine. Trust and communication are essential either way.

What if my child uses the potty at school but not at home?

If your child uses the potty at school but not at home, he may be trying to "push your buttons," or he may simply like the structure of the school potty routine. You can reverse some of the strategies in the previous question to create a more "school-like" routine at home:

- Borrow potty tricks from your child's teacher.
- Use the same words and transition cues.
- Recreate a similar potty schedule.
- Have the teacher send home encouraging potty notes.
- Show your child that you and the teacher are one potty team.

If your child is staging a potty mini-protest, avoid the power struggle. Rest assured that he understands the potty process and he's trying to incite an emotional reaction. Use a little humor to sidestep the conflict while letting him know you see the game. For example, make a silly nametag that says "Ms. So-and-So" and pretend you're the teacher and home is school. The goal is not necessarily to get your child to potty at home but for the two of you to laugh together at the silliness of going potty at school but not at home. Your child will start using the potty at home when it's no longer an emotionally charged game.

Is it ever okay to lie to my child about potty training?

Of course, honesty is the best practice. You certainly don't want to be caught in a lie. You lose months of trust-building if your child finds a package of perfectly good pull-ups after you say you don't have any more. You can't have it both ways—claim you don't have any, but secretly have a few just in case your bluff doesn't work. You can't say the school rule is all children must be potty trained and then have your child discover her new school friend doesn't have a potty clue.

One of the beauties of parenthood, though, is that you create a large part of your child's reality. As with all power, if used wisely, you might get away with it. Just like the car that won't start unless everyone has their seat belts on, the "lie" works if you always check seat belts before starting the car.

Ideally, a potty training lie is good if it is used to build your child's confidence, not if it is used to trick your child. Sometimes a cautious child must take the step forward before she knows she can do it. Your "lie" might show your child she can do something she never believed possible.

You might first try to translate the "lie" into a clear honest message. Maybe you won't have to lie at all. You can say, "Your teacher and I talked and we want you to wear your underpants this week—we think you can do it and we want you to try." Sometimes honesty is easier.

Is it okay to push my child if I know he's ready?

Should you buy a lottery ticket if you know you will win? Of course, you should. And potty training would be infinitely easier if you knew the future. Unfortunately, "pushing" your child is a gamble.

You can give your child a gentle "push" if he is truly ready in all areas of development. He is in control of his body and can hold his pee and poop until he gets to a potty. He sincerely wants to use the potty because it's important to him, not just because it's important to his parents, to school, or to anyone else. He has the social and the verbal skills to be successful in various potty situations, not just when the potty team orchestrates his success. He will be so proud of himself when he can finally say good-bye to diapers—and he won't look back with sadness or regret when he does. Your "push" is just what he needs to experience the final "aha." Then he will know, "Yes, I can do it!"

He is the child with the slow-to-warm-up temperament who wants to guarantee success before he takes a risk. He is the child with the difficult temperament who has trouble letting go until there are no other options. He is the child who needs a hand to hold before jumping into something new. He is the child who has a best friend standing right behind him stopping him from a turn-and-run. Your "push" is the ultimate act of trust.

Too often, however, the "push" is because someone else decides the child is ready. Usually, the child "can" potty but for whatever reason doesn't want to or chooses not to. If you "push" and your child does not want to be "pushed," you will set off a negative power struggle and an unnecessary battle of wills. Don't do it—it's not worth it!

How can I encourage my child to talk about a potty problem?

Potty-age children do not always know the right words to express emotions and problems. They have difficulty expressing themselves when they are confused, frustrated, or overwhelmed. You can feel like you're playing a guessing game—is it this or is it that? You might feel increasingly anxious if the situation concerns a change in your child's potty habits or a fear about a situation away from home.

If you want to encourage your child to talk about a potty situation, start by setting up good listening conditions and then help your child find the words that fit her needs. Children's concerns tend to percolate up at unexpected quieter times.

- Create listening times throughout the day when your child has your full attention—in the car, on walks, on a swing, at bedtime.
- Lead with open-ended statements—"I noticed you needed two changes of clothes at school today."
- Create a supportive environment for any possible answer, from "I hate school" to "You're stupid."
- Respond to feelings, not merely to words—"Sounds like it was a rough day" or "I can

help when you want to tell me about it."

- Don't rush—stay available to finish the conversation when your child is ready.
- Collect accurate information from other sources and tell your child what you think is happening—"The doctor says you need some medicine to help you poop. I want you to tell me when it hurts so I can help make it better."

What if my child is hesitant about asking other adults for potty help?

Your child's world is growing larger and larger all the time. It may include visits with family, playdates, or days at school. Your child may need your help learning to speak up for what he needs in a timely way. Even kindergartners can struggle with this one.

- Encourage your child to speak up at home. Resist the urge to read his mind just to save time. Verbalizing potty needs is an essential skill.
- Practice speaking up with different adults that your child knows. A child might hesitate to speak up because an adult looks or acts differently. A teacher might have different glasses or a quirky smile. Sometimes

adults appear gruff or rushed when in fact they are willing to help.

- Rehearse speaking with puppets or practicing with you. Be sure to let your child "play" himself and "play" the role of the other person.

- Be a positive role model. Let your child see you talking with the person. If the other person isn't a good listener, demonstrate how to catch that person's attention.

- Speak up. When you drop off your child in a new setting, let the other person know that your child needs some extra encouragement with this new skill.

How can I help if my child has an embarrassing potty experience in public or at school?

If you are with your child, treat a public potty accident with the same four-step protocol of Chapter 5, without too much high drama. Do not let your embarrassment contribute to your child's shame. If you happen to be in a non-child-friendly place, be prepared to neutralize negative stares and whispers with simple comments that your child can understand. "Yes, we had an accident and we're doing a good job of fixing the problem." Transform the negative moment into a family story to be retold often—"Remember the time you had the potty accident at the mall and everyone was looking at us…"

Sometimes a child might be leery of returning to the scene of a potty accident. Encourage her to return as soon as possible. If she's worried that an adult will scold her or children will laugh at her, give her the tools to face those situations. Speak to the adults in advance. Ask them to talk to your child immediately and explain they will not "be mean." Clarify what your child should do next time to avoid similar mistakes and ask for their help.

Plan a response with your child about how to face her peers. Help her choose her words—something strong and direct like, "Don't laugh at me. I don't like it and I wouldn't laugh at you." Enlist the help of the teacher for moral support. You cannot promise your child that people will be kind, but you can be ready to congratulate and comfort her.

How do we resume potty training after a setback (vacation, new sibling, new school, divorce)?

Your life may have been crazy for the last few months, but now you are ready to settle into a more child-focused potty training time. Chances are your child will be happy to be the center of attention again after all the other family excitement. Put out your potty "antennae" to see if your child is interested now. If not, the first step is to generate interest about a truly fun potty adventure.

- Get ready with your songs, games, and positive potty routines.
- Throw out a few gentle reminders—"We've been so busy ____, now we have time to think about the potty again."
- Use humor. Be dramatic—"One week with your grandparents and look what happens! Let's try those pull-ups again now that you're home and ready."
- Emphasize the fun potty experiences but still have no specific potty expectations. Follow your child's interest.
- Reschedule a "Potty Weekend" or "Naked Noons" when your child seems ready and interested. Otherwise, keep building interest in other positive ways.

What are the co-parenting strategies when parents absolutely disagree about the potty training plan?

Sometimes, no matter how much you try to stick to one consistent potty plan, both parents do not agree. Hopefully, you sincerely tried. If you tried everything short of marriage counseling and you must agree to disagree, here are a few important parenting guidelines. You want to maintain an atmosphere of mutual respect even when you agree to disagree. These strategies also apply to parents and grandparents, parents and teachers, and anyone who shares responsibility for raising a child.

1. Whoever speaks first is in charge of the situation. If one parent is playing potty games when the other parent thinks the child should be in bed, the parent in charge is the one who started the interaction with the child. It doesn't matter at this moment who is right or wrong. What matters is that one parent doesn't criticize the other parent in front of the child. The parent-in-charge gets to finish whatever was started. The other parent is free to go for a walk or put on earphones.

2. Talk about potty training disagreements after the incident-in-question has passed and when your child is away or sleeping. It's always easier to talk

about disagreements after emotions have cooled down. Wait until you can speak calmly to continue. Focus on the potty training goal and your child's short-term successes. Make modifications because they work for your child, not necessarily because they work for the adults.

3. Children learn different "rules" for different situations. As long as you are consistent with yourself, your child will know what each of you expects and how to manage those expectations. Simply explain the differences to your child; for example, "When you go to the store with Daddy, you have to follow Daddy's rules."

You child will learn how to adapt to different people in the real world. And she won't play one parent against the other. Now, you've turned a parenting negative into a parenting positive.

How do I respond to criticism about my potty training methods?

Not everyone agrees with all your parenting choices. So, chances are they won't all agree with your personal potty plan. And like it or not, you will never change them. If your child has a unique potty routine that draws comments from others, or if you know you will be an object of criticism in a certain situation, have your response ready ahead of time. It's hard to come up with the perfect words when you're the brunt of criticism. Try something simple like, "Please try to respect my right to do things the way I think best."

Do not try to defend your potty training choices when you feel under attack. You aren't likely to be heard. Let the person know you will happily explain your potty choices at a better time or place.

Most importantly, separate the criticism and the emotional repercussions from your interactions with your child. You will be teaching your child the bigger lesson of how to maneuver in a world where people disagree.

When should I consult with a pediatrician about potty concerns?

Your pediatrician is a wonderful resource and ally on your potty training team with a wealth of medical and developmental information. Contact your pediatrician whenever you need reassurance to the eternal parenting question, "Is this normal?" Sometimes, you just need to ask. Don't struggle and worry alone.

Successful potty training requires many behavioral, social, and emotional skills. It also requires a healthy body. You know your child's body better than you know your own. Contact your pediatrician whenever you have questions about your child's health.

- Contact your pediatrician any time your child's potty habits change
  - If your child is constipated
  - If your child starts having regular wetting accidents after months of success
  - If you notice small leaks regularly on underwear
- Contact your pediatrician if you notice changes in your child's pee or poop
  - Color (not food related)
  - Odors
  - Blood
  - Too hard or too soft
- Contact your pediatrician any time you suspect it's painful for your child to pee or to poop
- Contact your pediatrician anytime your child shows unexplainable physical distress
  - Fever
  - Vomiting
  - Refusal to eat
  - Lethargy
  - Abdominal or back pain
- Contact your pediatrician for bed wetting after the age of five or six

Chapter 8

READY TO GO

- When are we finished potty training?
- When should I put away all the potty props?
- How do I answer the inevitable question: "Where does the pee and poop go?"
- How should I respond to inappropriate potty talk?
- How do I respond to "peeing contests"?
- How can I tell if my child is manipulating me at bedtime with potty requests?
- When is my child ready for a sleepover?
- How do I plan for successful home sleepovers?
- How do I prevent bathroom lock-outs?
- How do I handle taking my opposite gender child into public bathrooms?
- When can my child go into a public bathroom alone?
- What do I do if there's no bathroom in sight?
- What has my child learned about his body during the pottying process?
- What has my child learned about learning?
- What have you learned from potty training?

When are we finished potty training?

Potty training started long before you set a date and time for your "Potty Plan." And it continues for a time after your child starts wearing underwear on a regular basis. You will use your "potty sense" for months, if not years, thinking for two and unconsciously being aware of bathrooms and bathroom stops. After all, accidents may happen when your child is excited, is in a new environment, or gets distracted during a fun activity.

Keep that extra bag of clothes in the back of the car through kindergarten. Many preschoolers have potty accidents. Sometimes, kindergartners have potty accidents. Plus, children are messy. A melting ice cream mess might be more likely than a potty accident. However, you'll be prepared if your child has an embarrassing accident. Speak to an older child with respectful sensitivity. Blame and shame are no more appropriate with an older child than with a younger child. Your older child is more verbal and can probably explain the source of her distress if asked gently. You can then problem solve a solution together.

The day always comes when you realize you aren't asking about your child's potty needs or giving any more reminders. Your child did it! She isn't wearing a pull-up to college.

You did it, too. Congratulations!

When should I put away all the potty props?

Potty chairs, travel potty seats, changing tables, diaper pails—good riddance! As your child grows into a little person, your home becomes less babyish. Every parent and child feels different things about the changes.

Think back to the temperament styles. Some parents and children never look back—"See ya, don't need ya!" If you haven't used the potty props for a month, pack them away. Even if your child has accidents, you don't want to become prop dependent again.

Parents and children with slow-to-warm-up temperaments will want a transition time. They will enjoy a few days to prepare for the inevitable. Some children dislike surprises, though it's not uncommon that it takes months for them to notice the change. Tell your child you will be putting away the potty gear. You can plan a simple and sweet farewell ritual. You and your child can sing a favorite potty song while you put the potty chair in a cardboard box and tape it up. Use this time to congratulate your child on his success. He should be very proud of himself!

How do I answer the inevitable question: "Where does the pee and poop go?"

The simple answer to your future engineer is: The pee and poop move from your house through pipes and they go back into the ground to add good things to the soil and the water. Zealous parents can really encourage a child's curiosity by planning a field trip with friends to the local water treatment plant. Children love seeing firsthand "where the poop goes."

Potty training is a study in self-discovery and in the biology of all living things. You could "study" in your own backyard what happens to animal and bug poop and pee. Young children love talking about poop and pee—start watching for "evidence" on neighborhood walks. If you have a dog, let your child hose the poops and watch them disappear into the ground. If you're on a walk and scoop the dog poop in a bag, put it in a garbage can and talk about what happens next. Birds, snails, raccoons—the investigation is limitless and definitely interesting to a young child.

How should I respond to inappropriate potty talk?

Your child is the master of the bathroom and of her body. She has also learned the power of potty words—poopy head, pee pee breath, penis face, and every combination thereof. The words have power because children laugh and adults go wild. The behavior is all about attention. As soon as you remove the pay-off, the behavior will disappear.

As always, remove the emotional incentive. Your child has the "power" if she knows she is pushing your buttons. It is better for her to discover that power through her other positive abilities. Speak calmly and directly: "I don't like those words." If your child continues, remove the audience. Leave the scene or separate the children. Again, explain what you're doing: "We aren't going to listen to you," or "We'll be back when you're done being silly."

Calm and direct always works. There are some situations, however, when your child isn't sure you mean what you say. In these cases, the provocative behavior escalates. Stay calm. Your child is just checking you.

Of course, you are human. If your first reaction was to hush, scold, and threaten, that's normal. Just take three steps backwards—admit that you lost it, explain again calmly what behavior is appropriate, and change the immediate situation. Let it be— there's no need to repeat your point until your child winds up for a second round.

How do I respond to "peeing contests"?

Whether it's Freud or testosterone, boys discover quickly that penises can pee near and far, in lines and in circles, on walls or on snow. This gets to be a problem when you realize your child has inadvertently crossed your comfort boundary. While your child's actions begin as spontaneous and innocent, they can quickly pass the line of what you consider appropriate.

Teach your child appropriate behaviors early—what's okay outside but not inside, what's okay in the back yard but not in the front yard, what's okay at home with Dad but not at school or at friends' houses.

- Know your child. Your boundaries might be realistic or unrealistic. Keep the rules simple if you think your child will have difficulty remembering them.
- Know the power of peers. Expect the laughter and attention of peers to outweigh the most sensible rules.
- Know the principle of escalating action. Some actions are so completely self-satisfying that they assume their own momentum. Know when to stop and when to continue before behavior gets out of control.

How can I tell if my child is manipulating me at bedtime with potty requests?

Children learn quickly that parents will jump at the promise of potty success. Call it potty power. However, potty requests should not take priority over your bedtime routine. A request for "One more," and then "One more," should be answered with "Last time." Nighttime potty training is about your child's ability to empty her bladder before bedtime and then wait until morning. If your child had a little more to drink and needs to use the potty, she knows how to take care of those needs without your participation.

Establish a clear, consistent nighttime routine—one trip to the potty, never more than two. If your child calls your bluff and has an accident, clean it up calmly and return her to bed as quickly as possible. Resist the urge for any potty discussions at this time. Tomorrow night, watch your child's intake of liquids, stay with the bedtime routine, and remind your child that this is the last potty stop for the night. Therefore, she should let all the pee out now.

Your child may spend a few nights trying to engage you in a potty power play. The challenge will end when she is convinced that you mean what you say. The other scenario has you waiting for her bathroom calls for months.

When is my child ready for a sleepover?

Potty training is not a prerequisite skill for a happy sleepover. If your child is comfortable at a relative's house or at a friend's house, he can have a successful sleepover. You just need good communication and a realistic plan.

Give your child's host an accurate description of his potty skills.

- Be completely honest with your child. If your child has accidents, don't let him talk you into believing he won't. He can go on the sleepover if he agrees to realistic conditions.

- Make a realistic plan. Do you need the host to be a hands-on potty helper? Does your child need to agree to nighttime pull-ups? Do you need to send along a plastic mattress cover or your child's sleeping bag?

- Be completely honest about what's required for success. If the host doesn't want to be responsible to give your child reminders, it is better to wait a few months or longer to find a more appropriate sleepover host.

- Give it a try and have a Plan B just in case:
  - Prepare in your head—"If this doesn't work, I'm ready to give a great pep talk and we'll go to our favorite place for breakfast."

- Arrange with your child—"If you have an accident, I'll pack extra pajamas and your friend's mom will wrap up your sleeping bag for you."
- Discuss in advance with the host— "If you notice that my son is upset, please call me at any time. I'll be happy to pick him up."

How do I plan for successful home sleepovers?

If sleeping away from home is uncomfortable for your child, invite your child's friends to a sleepover at your house. Respect your child's preference to either be open and nonchalant about her potty skills or to be quiet and discreet. Discretion is fine, but be sure your child is getting positive messages in your home that nighttime accidents are normal.

- Talk to your child ahead of time if she wears nighttime pull-ups. Is she okay that her friends see her pull-ups or does she want to put them on privately?
- Create a positive nighttime potty routine. It is better to do your "mom act" than have your child pretend not to need her usual bathroom routine.

- Incorporate the games for middle-of-the-night trips to the bathroom.
- Design sleeping arrangements to fit the situation—plastic mattress covers, sleeping bags, camping cots, and a camping theme.
- Have an accident plan. Don't ask children to guess what they should do "if," especially in an emotionally sensitive situation. Tell them you are nearby and ready to help.
- Plan a response to teasing, just in case. You never know if another child might say something hurtful. Teach your child early that those hurtful words say more about the speaker than about her. Remind her of "the truth" that potty accidents are nothing to be ashamed of. Then, teach her to stand up for herself and to tell others to "stop saying hurtful words."

How do I prevent bathroom lock-outs?

While your child is young, make it a practice to keep the bathroom door open. If your child requests "privacy," tell him he may close the door when an adult is with him. Water, glass, and hard surfaces make bathrooms potentially dangerous. Open doors allow you to supervise any possible bathroom play.

Your potty trained child's curiosity might be tempted by the extra bathroom time. Check your bathroom door locks before your child realizes he can lock you out. Turn the handle around so the lock is on the outside of the door—that way, no one can get locked in. Replace knobs that have locks with simple handles, or keep keys to the bathroom door in an accessible place. Popping the bathroom door off the hinges is time consuming if you are trying to get to your child quickly.

How do I handle taking my opposite gender child into public bathrooms?

Family restrooms and single-toilet bathrooms make parents' lives much easier. Both parents can co-parent, venturing separately into the world with their children.

When faced with a men's room and a ladies' room, however, moms have a distinct advantage. Since the baby changing stations are in the women's rest room, moms with little boys can do what they always did— bring boys into the ladies' room. If a mom wants her son to experience the urinal in the men's bathroom, she should go into the bathroom with her child. It's probably best to announce your entrance before coming through the door, "Mom coming in!"

Dads can do the same when entering a ladies'
bathroom, "Dad coming in!" More typically, dads are
taking daughters into the men's room. Rumor has it
that men's rooms might not be as clean and potty-
friendly as the ladies' rooms. You might consider
packing your child's backpack with sanitizing wipes,
toilet seat covers, or a travel potty seat. Some dads
choose to avoid the decision altogether and carry a
travel potty.

When can my child go into a public bathroom alone?

Young children should not go into public bathrooms
without supervision. Although your child might enjoy
the freedom of pottying on her own, that doesn't
mean she is old enough to be alone in a public bathroom. Young children do not have the cognitive skills
to predict negative consequences and they cannot
know the risks inherent in certain decisions. Even
when children have been taught safety routines, they
are easily distracted and persuaded to act otherwise.
Adults, not children, are responsible for keeping children safe. Besides, if they go into a bathroom alone,
who will be there to watch your child's hand washing?

There is no reason not to accompany your child
into a public bathroom. However, if you choose to

wait outside a public bathroom door for your child, create a bathroom game that keeps you in contact with your child. Play "Daddy echo," repeating silly things that your child says or an alphabet/counting game where each one of you says the next letter/number.

What do I do if there's no bathroom in sight?

If time runs out and you're on a busy city street, you may not have many options. Do whatever you can to minimize your child's discomfort and to make clean-up as easy as possible. Don't waste a lot of breath on "woulda, coulda, shoulda." Just remember your four-step accident response—1. Check your emotions, 2. Describe the problem, 3. Find a solution, and 4. End with a positive.

If you are lucky enough to be outdoors near a tree or a bush, it's time for potty au naturel. Boys, of course, can be far more discreet than girls, and the outside world offers wonderful new objects for the aim game. Girls will need your help to avoid wetting their clothes. Show them how to squat, help them with balance, and try to anticipate their aim—watch out for their shoes. Hopefully you will have some tissues and a zipper baggie to carry them to the trash.

The outdoor experience can be liberating and fun for many children. So, if you plan on limiting pottying outdoors, be prepared to explain the "rules" immediately. You may want your child to ask permission first or one day you might catch him peeing on Aunt Cathy's rose bushes.

What has my child learned about his body during the pottying process?

Potty training brings together body, mind, and emotions at a time when your child is becoming an independent person. He is now in control of his body and is capable of taking care of an important physical need every day. He can enjoy the pride of his accomplishment. You, meanwhile, can enjoy a newfound freedom from diapers.

Continue to support a healthy connection between your child's body and mind. Your child learned his body is predictable and gives him clear signals about what it needs. Build on your child's awareness that he knows his body. Whether he's tired, hungry, or sleepy, let him "read" his body just like he does when he needs to potty. Guide him to choices that will honor his body. Then, he will grow up knowing that his body and his mind work together to make him happy and healthy.

What has my child learned about learning?

Potty training might have been easy or challenging. Either way, your child learned about learning. She mastered a complex skill that leads the way to new freedom and independence. She learned to take responsibility for her needs and her actions. She learned to trust others to guide her to good choices and to ask for help when she needs it. She learned to take a few risks in new situations, that it was better to take a risk and make a mistake than to take no risk at all. She learned that learning eventually leads to success.

In retrospect, she is both the same child you held in your arms a few years ago and a different child who has new needs and abilities. Every time your child passes a new developmental milestone, she grows. Most of all, your child learned she is smart, capable, and loved.

What have you learned from potty training?

Potty training is an important milestone in your child's development. Potty training is also a huge milestone in the stages of parent development. Much has been written about parent–infant bonding, but you just went through an extraordinary "dance" of mutual cooperation. When your child was an infant, you tuned into his likes, dislikes, and needs, large and small. You anticipated how to make him happy and minimize his distress and discomfort. You created a world of love and belonging just for him.

In potty training, you did the same dance but this time your child was an active partner. You learned your child's strengths and your child's limits. You taught your child to trust those strengths and to face those limits—to use one and to rise above the other. You created a potty training world for your child to try, to fail, and to succeed. You learned when to lead and when to follow. Potty training is a success that you share with your child.

In every case, you also learned something about yourself as a parent. You may have discovered a few unknown strengths—resilience, humor, patience— along with a few personal limits—frustration, confusion, despair. But you grew with your child. You are not exactly the same person you were when you began this potty adventure, but you are definitely better equipped for the next stage of parenting.

Chapter 9

REAL
MOMENTS—
SPECIFIC
QUESTIONS
FROM THE
TRENCHES

- What do I do when my child wants to use the potty, tries to use the potty, but nothing happens?
- What do I do when my child has been successfully using a potty training sticker chart and then loses interest?
- What do I do when my potty trained child regresses after one week away with grandparents?
- What do I do when my child walks to the potty and then poops in the diaper?
- What do I do when my child dislikes wet diapers but has no interest in the potty?
- What do I do when my child wants to use the potty but is fearful of the potty?
- What do I do when my child has been trained for months and regresses when a parent starts to travel for business?
- What do I do when my child holds the pee when on the potty and then immediately goes in the diaper?
- What do I do when my child is potty trained but still wants to wear a diaper?
- What do I do when my daughter imitates males when peeing?
- What do I do when I think my child is manipulating me?
- What do I do when my child wants to potty train with only one person?

- ■ What do I do when my child has accidents at school because he wants me to come to school?
- ■ What do I do when my child's school doesn't want to use our potty seat?
- ■ What do I do when I think my child is potty trained but lazy?

My son tells me he has to go to the potty and I take him. All he does is sit there and ask for toilet paper. I do see him squeezing his belly muscles like he's trying to make something happen, but it never does. I feel bad and I don't want to discourage him from the potty, but I don't have all day to sit with him.

Here's a situation where you can see obvious readiness in some areas but not in all. Your son has the intellectual readiness (knows what to do on the potty) and the emotional readiness (he has the desire), but he doesn't have the physical readiness to make it happen when he wants. Unfortunately, until that last piece of the puzzle is in place, you could be waiting in the bathroom all day—which is not the best use of your time, or his.

You can encourage him by following his lead. Support his interest and let him sit on the potty, ready or not. Make a big deal of looking to see if pee or poop came out. If not, tell him "Oh well—maybe next time." Continue the positive potty routine—wipe with toilet paper, flush the toilet, wash hands, and pull up pants.

If you notice your son looking like he might have to potty, explain what that feels like and that this is a good time to sit on the potty. You can point to the place on his body where he feels it. There's absolutely no hurry. Your son is a smart boy and this will all make sense to him in no time.

We had a sticker chart with a reward system that my daughter was really into when we first started. Now, she's just not interested in it anymore.

One of the problems with stickers is that they lose their effectiveness when the novelty wears off. They are fun at first because they are new and children love the attention. Sticker charts are meaningful when they support your child's interest versus when the charts are intended to generate interest. For example, if your child is striving to be potty proficient, the sticker chart is a concrete record of getting closer and closer to her goal.

Smart children, who are not potty motivated, realize fairly early that they have other options. This creates an opportunity for a power struggle—similar to when you offer your child a choice of "blue" or "red" and your child picks "green." At some point, your child figures out that it's not about stickers at all but about something else that she doesn't really want to do. And she rebels.

Honor her choice and wait on the potty training until she has an interest that will sustain her through the training process. You will enjoy it more and so will she.

My little girl is two-and-a-half and we potty trained her Memorial Day weekend. It took four days of accidents and she's been dry as a bone and doing terrifically. We sent her up to New York City with the grandparents for a week for the Fourth of July, and since she came back she hasn't had one dry day yet. I don't know what to do, it's been very frustrating and I'm upset. I know she is capable of staying dry because for practically two whole months she was.

Ambivalence is a powerful emotion. You may not expect to see it so strongly in two-and-a-half-year-olds. Of course, it's part of emotional growth. Two-year-olds want it all: I want to grow up—I don't want to grow up. I like the potty—I miss my diaper. I want to take care of myself—I want my mommy to take care of me. Potty training is easy—Potty training is work. Potty-age children get stuck in the contradictions and then regress to the old comfort zone.

Another explanation is that the grandparents could have relaxed the potty routine. Maybe they were too busy playing and laughing with their granddaughter to think about skill building. If so, it's a very temporary setback. Travel and a week away could also disrupt your daughter's potty routine. Time with grandparents is worth far more than uninterrupted potty training.

Take a step back for the next few weeks, without any potty expectations whatsoever. During those two weeks, talk with your daughter about how easy it was for both of you when she used the potty. Remind your daughter that she was happy and successful and wore those pretty underpants. Make a joke about "Then you went to visit your grandparents and look what happened." Be dramatic. Throw your hands up in the air.

Eliminate any negative emotional judgments on your part. Her potty "rebellion" is her choice, not a power struggle. Set the stage to get back to a positive potty experience. She did it before—she will do it again.

My twenty-month-old daughter has started telling me when she is ready to poop. Several times she has walked over to her potty, sat down on it, and said, "Poop, poop, poop," and then proceeded to go in her diaper. She has not done this regarding "Pee pee"; however, she does seem to hold her pee and let it out all at once. Is it time to start officially potty training?

It's tempting to see a few of the early readiness signs and want to start more structured potty training. Usually children under two years old are still months away from potty independence. Your daughter may start pooping on the potty regularly, or she may not. If she is going to pee on the potty, she needs a very hands-on potty partner for the next six to eight months. You can start now and invest a lot of time, or you can wait six months and invest a few weeks.

This is, however, a perfect time to follow your daughter's lead and celebrate the connection she's made between her body and her potty chair. Talk about body parts and pottying. Talk about what it feels like when she goes pee and poop, and then talk about what it feels like before she goes pee and poop.

The feeling before and the desire to hold it for a special place are essential.

Be a positive potty role model. Incorporate a few potty success times; for example, before bath time. With a fun and interesting potty environment, you will be more likely to notice your daughter staying dry for longer periods of time. Then, you'll be ready to kick off your "Personal Potty Plan."

My son is twenty-seven-months old and very unhappy when his diaper leaks, but he has shown no interest in sitting on the potty. He doesn't seem to care about potty training at all, and we are expecting our second child next month. Your child is still missing the motivational readiness to begin a structured potty program. And with a new baby arriving soon, you don't need to add anything else to your soon-to-be-even-busier schedule. Your son's next few months should be focused on welcoming the baby and becoming a big brother.

Since your son has noticed that he doesn't like the feel of the leaky diaper, casually use that information to create new awareness. Explain that it's the pee that feels funny and one day he will know when the pee is ready to come out. Tell him to let you know if he gets a pee-pee feeling.

Motivation will follow cognitive awareness. As you go about your normal routine, talk about everyone's potty experience—Mom, Dad, and especially the new baby. Talk about diapers and underpants. Let your son, of course, help change the baby—bring the diapers, sprinkle the powder. Let him know that he knows things about his body that the baby won't know for years. Build the positive potty connections and your son's self-awareness. After the baby settles into an easy routine, your son will probably be ready to explore his new potty options.

My daughter will be three years old in six weeks. She is petrified of the toilet! She talks big, talks about going on the potty and wearing big-girl underpants (which we have in every character sold in stores!). However, once she gets undressed and approaches the potty, she cries and resists our attempts to get her sitting on it. She has actually "gone" on the potty twice so far. Once she peed and once she pooped, but she

refuses to go on anymore. I am at a loss. Peer pressure doesn't seem to affect her in this arena and I don't know what to try next!

Your brave little daughter has tried to "talk" herself into feeling comfortable around the potty. Of course, she can't and her feelings of panic escalate. She has the cognitive readiness to use the potty. She probably even has the physical control. But without the emotional confidence, she will continue to be overwhelmed. Tell her sincerely that you don't want her to be sad or worried about going on the potty—there's no hurry.

Encourage her to verbalize her experience. If sitting on the potty upsets her, tell her to say, "I don't want to sit on the potty right now." As a three-year-old, your daughter probably has the language skills to speak up for what she wants and needs.

Work on building her emotional comfort. Tell her not to sit on the potty naked for now. Try having her sit on it with her clothes on. Ask questions that will focus her attention on a positive potty experience and not on the fears—"Do you like the little potty or the big potty?" "Is the potty seat like a circle or like a square?" Try building confidence through playful experiences—using books, dolls, or songs. She needs to rehearse her skills in easy settings before practicing for "real."

Do everything you can to help your daughter feel in control of the potty experience. When she feels strong and capable, the rest will be easy.

My daughter has been potty trained for six months. But when I started traveling for my job, my daughter regressed completely. Nothing works. I tried telling her she's past that, tried bringing her presents, tried taking away privileges. She seems happy as can be to be back in diapers.

Separation strategies take priority over potty training strategies. When your daughter insists on a diaper, it might be a way to stay "in control" of a situation she can't control. Try some games and routines to help your child adjust to the changes in your schedule first and then reestablish a positive potty routine.

Give your child something tangible to help her comprehend when you're coming and when you're going—a calendar with heart stickers when you're home and star stickers when you're in a hotel under the stars. Establish a phone call routine when you read a bedtime story or sing a bedtime song. Create a travel rhyme she can say when she misses you: "Mommy, Mommy (or Daddy, Daddy) far away...have a great big awesome day," and blow kisses. Give the new routine a few weeks to settle in.

Accept your daughter's potty preference without overreacting. Keep providing simple, positive potty routines. Your daughter will regain her physical and emotional equilibrium in no time.

My son sits on the potty and says he doesn't have to go. As soon as we put him back in his diaper, he goes in the diaper. I know he can control it.

There's a difference between him "knowing he can control it" and him deciding where he wants to release it. In this case, his intention is different than your intention. Since this is his body, he wins.

He is exerting self-control by waiting for the diaper. Build on his need for independence. Explain that you noticed he is choosing to go in the diaper and give your permission to still wear the diaper sometimes. Try to engage his participation in other aspects of the potty process so he is taking responsibility even though he is still relying on the diapers. He will soon discover he doesn't need the comfort of the diaper.

Remember, urgency on your part often means stress and resistance on your child's part. Acknowledge his fear of "letting go," balance emotional support and practical support, and be flexible to allow him to conquer the problem in his own time.

My child insists on wearing a diaper even though he is completely potty trained. He simply takes off his diaper or asks to be changed but he pees and poops in the potty. I've tried everything, buying fun underwear, putting underwear over the diaper, but he insists he does not want to give up the diaper.

Some children have strong emotional attachments to their diapers. Keep things low key to prevent an escalating power struggle. Affirm the positive—"I know one day you'll tell me when you want to wear your underwear." Indeed, he will decide one day that he's has enough time with diapers.

You can also try the ABC response here. Acknowledge your child's preference. Say something light-hearted but without sarcasm, "You're the first child I know who uses the potty but still likes to wear a diaper." You want him to know that you accept his choice at this time.

Balance your response between comfort and power. Try to verbalize what he thinks are the advantages of diapers over underwear. Talk about the diapers having soft thick padding whereas underwear is made of thin material. Experiment with short intervals in underwear if he agrees. Sing the "Big Underwear" song by Joe Scruggs.

If your child is young and the diaper isn't creating any problems at school, your child will conquer this problem in his own time. The awareness of same-age peers is also a natural incentive. However, if you believe your child needs your help because the diaper is increasingly a source of embarrassment or frustration, slowly prepare him for a change. Let him know that on a particular day, you aren't buying any more diapers. Let your child participate in a countdown to the date by marking off calendar days or by seeing the number of diapers get smaller and smaller. Then he can prepare himself for the inevitable leap into underwear.

My daughter stands and pees while holding her imaginary penis.

Parents should keep a potty training diary of all the funny and unique things their children do. Your daughter must have some wonderful male role models. Don't let her catch you laughing at her and don't let her hear you telling others, but enjoy, enjoy, enjoy.

If she struggles with the logistics of standing and peeing, you can tell her that daddies and brothers stand because they have penises and mommies and sisters sit because they have vaginas. Otherwise, let this be the beginning of countless gender biases she will single-handedly overturn.

I think my five-year-old daughter is manipulating me. She's old enough to wipe herself after pooping but she says she can't do it and wants me to wipe her.

Your daughter may be manipulating you or she may have a genuine emotional need. Here's another situation where the ABC response can help de-escalate a negative situation and support your daughter's emotional growth and personal responsibility. If you react with a harsh "No, you do it yourself," the emotional tug-of-war can spiral out of control. She will be collapsing on the floor in whiney pleas of "Help meeeee." You will catapult into doubt, "Should I help—shouldn't I help?" And the drama continues.

Instead, calmly acknowledge the problem by saying, "I know you think you need me but I want you to learn how to wipe yourself." Then, balance your emotional support with your practical support. For example, "I'll stay here while you wipe. Let me see you try." Depending on your child's intensity level, she may be able to try to succeed or she may attempt to prove to you that she can't succeed. Try not to get frustrated as you watch her attempts. Instead, evaluate where her frustration is coming from. If it is a learned helplessness, empower her with small successes and gentle encouragement. If it's attention-getting behavior, check your negative emotional reaction and give positive attention in other appropriate situations. Ambivalent emotions about growing up and staying small show up repeatedly during developmental growth spurts.

The ability, "I know she can do it herself," is only half the equation for success. Your child has to believe it, too. She conquers the problem when she learns how to act responsibly without the emotional overtures. You are teaching skills as well as confidence and personal pride.

I have a little boy with my second husband and two older children from a previous marriage. I am in the midst of potty training my son with little success. I know he is capable as he has been successful when he's with my thirteen-year-old daughter. Should I allow her to participate in the training and step aside or should I persevere until he is willing to cooperate with me?

Young children have many creative ways of taking control of their potty experiences. One way or another, they have to do it "their way." Luckily, you have a thirteen-year-old on your potty team. She probably brings fun and patience to training process. If your thirteen-year-old is willing, keep her actively involved. But do not "step aside." Your ultimate goal is to build independence from any one routine.

Use the ABC response to respect your son's preferences and to gradually introduce more flexibility. Acknowledge your son's "game." "I know you like your sister helping." Be sincere, "You are lucky to have a big sister who loves you and wants to teach you so many things."

Balance your response between accepting where your child is at this moment in time and creating a bridge to your final goal. Emphasize the positive potty experience and try to recreate the positives with other people. When your older daughter is not available for potty time, she can encourage your son to be successful without her. Be sure she checks on his progress and celebrates any successes he has with other people.

Your son will conquer this problem when he lets go of his need to control his potty team. Your son has to agree to a potty plan when his sister is unavailable. You can guide that choice according to what works for you—Is he willing to go to the potty without her? Is he willing to accept your help? Does he want to wear his diaper? Once he sees that the choice is his, he will have the control he's fighting for and can go back to enjoying the pride of potty mastery with or without his sister.

My son's school calls the parents to change poopy diapers in preschool-age children. I think my son is having accidents because he wants me to come to the school, not because he can't remember to use the potty.

Discuss the possibility of a separation issue both with your son and with the school. Address the separation issue separate from the potty issue. You should plan fun activities for the two of you immediately after school. Talk to your son's teacher about in-school separation strategies—love-notes in his lunchbox, a laminated heart for his pocket, and so on. Read Audrey Penn's book *The Kissing Hand* and incorporate a special farewell kiss into your morning routine. Try to fulfill your son's separation needs in new positive ways.

With the cooperation of the school, leave a change of clothes and enlist someone from the school to change your son in the event of an accident. If the school cannot compromise school policy to change your son, recruit another friend or family member to go to the school in your place. Focus on the positive— telling your son that you want him to be successful and enjoy all the wonderful things at school.

My child is doing well with potty training using a child's potty seat on our home toilet. I would like there to be consistency in my child's potty experience from home to school, but school policy is that parents cannot bring potty props to school.

School is one of the first steps you and your child

take into the world outside of your family. While you will share many similarities in educational philosophy, you will also experience some practical differences in day-to-day situations. Schools set policies like these based on the logistics of managing groups of children and on their experience of what children are able to learn in a group setting.

Trust the school to help your child adjust to this change while she is there. You might be surprised that the flexibility she learns at school will carry over to home. Your child deserves your confidence that she can learn this new potty independence. Give her time to make the adjustment. She is also learning how to accept help from other caring people.

Although it is natural to want to protect your child from frustrations and difficulties, stay positive while she is in that limbo between the old and new ways. She will trust the school only if you do. Do not criticize the rule or the school in front of your child. Schedule a private conversation with the teacher or the director if you need reassurance or progress reports.

I think my child is just lazy. He was completely potty trained and uses the potty at school and when we're out. But at home, he doesn't care. He'll go on the potty when he wants to and other times he just goes in his pants.

The good news is that your child understands the potty process in public situations. He understands his body and he understands the expectations. Calling him "lazy" at home is counterproductive. You may feel frustrated and helpless, leading to no-win power struggles. Just because he "can" potty doesn't mean he "will" potty.

Talk to your son about the different choices he's making at home and away from home. Acknowledge that it's his choice but state calmly that you would like him to use the potty at home, too. Explain that life is easier when he uses the toilet all the time. Balance your response between emotions and problem solving. Does your son need emotional support with some new challenges in his world—a new school, a new sibling? If the accidents happen regularly, does he need to wear a pull-up until he is ready to take responsibility for his body at home?

Home may be a safe place for your son to regress. Potty training may not be your son's priority at the moment. Or, he may be too engaged in an activity to stop to potty. He will conquer the problem when you remove any negative attention that reinforces a power game, establish positive potty routines that remind him to take regular potty breaks, and allow him to catch up to fully enjoy his own successes.

POTTY BOOKS, VIDEOS, AND STORIES

Popular Children's Potty Books

A Potty for Me! by Karen Katz
Does a Pig Flush? by Fred Ehrlich
Everyone Poops by Taro Gomi
Go, Girl! Go Potty! by Harriet Ziefert Inc.
Going to the Potty by Fred Rogers
I Have to Go! by Robert Munsch
Lift the Lid, Use the Potty by Annie Ingle and Lisa McCue
No More Diapers for Ducky by Bernette Ford and Sam
   Williams
No Potty! Yes, Potty! by Harriet Ziefert Inc.
Once Upon a Potty by Alona Frankel
The Prince and the Potty by Wendy Cheyette Lewison
The Princess and the Potty by Wendy Cheyette
   Lewison
The Potty Book for Boys by Alyssa Satin Capucilli
The Potty Book for Girls by Alyssa Satin Capucilli
Time to Pee by Mo Willems

Uh Oh! Gotta Go! Potty Tales from Toddlers by Bob
   McGrath
What Do You Do with a Potty? by Marianne Borgardt
Where's the Poop? by Julie Markes and Susan
   Kathleen Hartung
You Can Go to the Potty by William Sears, MD,
   Martha Sears, RN, and Christie Watts Kelly
Your New Potty by Joanna Cole

Homemade Potty Books and Stories

My Potty Book—a personal "how to" potty chronicle
My Two Houses—a visual comparison of "new" and
   "old" potties
My World of Potties—a pictorial study of various toilets and potties
Underwear and Diapers—a book of friends and
   family and what they wear

Oral Storytelling

Fast Boy—the story of the child who can't sit still
Growing Every Day—the story of changing from a
   baby to a child
My Body and Me—the explanation of a child's body
   and feelings

Underwear Books

Arthur's Underwear by Marc Brown
Underwear! by Mary Elise Monsell and Lynn
  Munsinger
What Color Is Your Underwear? by Sam Lloyd

Favorite Children's Potty Videos

Bear in the Big Blue House by Martin Hugh Mitchell
I Can Go Potty by Mazzarella Productions
It's Potty Time by Learning Through Entertainment,
  Inc.
Let's Go Potty by Dr. Betti Hertzberg
Once Upon a Potty for Her by Alona Frankel
Once Upon a Potty for Him by Alona Frankel

Appendix B

POTTY SONGS, RHYMES, AND CDS

Children's Potty Songs and Music

Ants by Joe Scruggs ("Big Underwear")

Miss Joanie's Potty Party by Joanie Whittaker

The Once Upon a Potty—Potty Songs CD by Ari Frankel

Potty Animal: Funny Songs about Potty Training by Auntie Poo & The Porta-Potties

Potty Song: Customized Potty Training Song at www.pottysong.com

Potty Song 1, *Potty Song 2*, and *Potty Song 3* (free potty songs) at www.pottytrainingconcepts.com

Tinkle, Tinkle, Little Tot: Songs and Rhymes for Toilet Training (book) by Bruce Lansky, Robert Pottle, and Friends

Improvised Potty Songs
Happy Potty Song (Tune: "Happy Birthday")
Happy potty to me.

Happy potty to me.

I'm learning where to pee.

Happy potty to me!

Happy potty to me.

Happy potty to me.

I'm learning where to poopie.

Happy potty to me!

This Is The Way (Tune: "Here We Go 'Round the Mulberry Bush")
This is the way we sit on the potty,

Sit on the potty, sit on the potty,

This is the way we sit on the potty,

Early in the morning.

(every afternoon/early in the ev'ning/before we go to bed)

Are You Peeing? (Tune: "Frere Jacques")
Are you peeing? Are you peeing?

Little one? Little one?

Yes, I am. Yes, I am.

Now I'm done. Now I'm done.

Bathroom Clean-Up Song (Tune: "Old McDonald")

Substitute your child's name for David

Little David cleaned the mess.

E-I-E-I-O.

With a wipe wipe here and a wipe wipe there.

E-I-E-I-O.

Little David cleaned the mess.

E-I-E-I-O.

Additional Verses:

Little David sprayed the spray.

Little David wiped the floor.

Little David pitched the trash.

Appendix C POTTY TRAINING GAMES

Potty Time Signals

Draw a "P" with a question mark on your child's back.

Give a "T" hand signal for a potty time-out.

Set fun buzzers or timers.

Sitting on the Potty Games

Whistle while you wait.

Play "I spy."

Play "I hear."

Customize your own "Fast Boy" story.

Happy Successes

Potty tallies on a bathroom whiteboard or chalkboard

Happy faces on the bathroom mirror

Bathroom bell ringing

Mini-celebrations with cupcakes and a potty candle-lighting ceremony

A photo wall of happy potty pictures

Phone calls with positive potty reports to friends and relatives

"Red light" and "green light" cards

"High Five" wall poster

Toilet paper rolls for your child to "toot her horn"

Grand Finale Rituals

Dance around a trash can as you throw away the last diaper.

Throw an underwear party and have everyone wear silly underwear over their clothes,

fly underwear-wearing helium balloons, and invite friends and family to an underwear parade where they will be waving underwear on sticks.

Appendix D POTTY TRAINING RESOURCES

Potty Training Supplies

Potty seats and chairs

Potty toppers

Potty training car seat liners

Step stools

Potty training pants and covers

Potty training dolls

Potty training charts and stickers

Potty training games and calendars

Potty time watches

Potty targets

Potty training urinals

Flushable potty clothes and wipes

Toilet paper for children

Mattress pads and covers

Night lights and toilet lights

Velcro easy-off belts

Potty travel mitts

Auto-flush stoppers
Potty training cleaning supplies

Potty Resource Websites

www.babycenter.com
www.babylove.com
www.babiesrus.com
www.companystore.com
www.pottytrainingconcepts.com
www.pottytrainingsolutions.com
www.onestepahead.com

Index

A
Accidents
  after success, 138
  belittling by others, 131
  changing clothes after, 144–45
  cleaning up, 131–32
  child self-esteem and, 147–48
  distractions and, 124
  emotions and, 125, 127–28
  as game, 127–28
  last minute-too late pottying, 135
  leaving potty too soon, 136
  likelihood of, 123–24
  natural consequences, 129–30
  nighttime, 141–43
  occurrence of, 122–23
  punishment vs. natural consequences, 130
  reaction to, 125–26
  scolding, 128–29
  too many, 145
Adoption, potty training during, 86–87
Adult temperament styles, 56–58
Afternoon mini-sessions, 74–76

V
Vegetables, 100
Verbal behaviors, 38
Verbal reminders, 134
Verbal strengths, of child, 112–13
Videos, 153–56, 253
Vocabulary choices, for body parts and bodily functions, 96–97

W
Water, 100
Websites, 177–78, 262
"Weekend Mini's", 70, 76–79, 105, 106–07
Weekend warrior parents, 72–73
Wheat bread, 100
Wiping, 24–25, 242–43
Withholding poop, 192–94
Words, for body parts and bodily functions, 96–97
Working parents, 73
Wrong method, 10–11

Y
"Yes" people, 73

About the Author

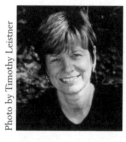

Photo by Timothy Leistner

Karen Deerwester is the owner of Family Time Coaching & Consulting and a highly requested speaker and trainer for parents and educators in South Florida. Karen reaches millions of parents each month as the parent expert for Bluesuitmom.com, the author of the Toddler/Preschooler Column for *South Florida Parenting* magazine and numerous parenting websites. Karen's popular parenting CD, *Parenting Quick Tips for Young Children*, was featured in the premiere issue of Dr. Phil's *The Next Level*.